Why Is There a Hammer in the
Fridge?

To
Teresa
Best of Luck

& Nora Trujillo

(Dr.t.) 10/26/13

Why Is There a Hammer in the Fridge?

A Family Member's Guide to Alzheimer's

Moraima Trujillo, MD
with Nora Trujillo

the
small
press

Why Is There a Hammer in the Fridge?
A Family Member's Guide to Alzheimer's

Brown Books Small Press
16250 Knoll Trail, Suite 205
Dallas, Texas 75248
www.BBSmallPress.com
(972) 381-0009

ISBN 978-1-61254-112-9
LCCN 2013940697

Printed in the United States of America
10 9 8 7 6 5 4 3 2 1

To my father, Esmeraldo Trujillo,
who always dreamed of helping others

Contents

Preface

It was painfully frustrating when no one could tell me what was wrong with my father. There is no substitute for being well informed about any disease. That is why I wrote this book. At the time that he first started showing symptoms of Alzheimer's, I couldn't find anyone who knew anything about what was wrong with my dad. So I resolved to educate myself. I haven't stopped learning and live convinced that education is key to helping those afflicted by this disease and their loved ones.

Acknowledgments

I would like to thank my daughter, Nora, for her contributions to this book; my father, for inspiring me to help others; and my patients, from whom I always learn more.

Thank you to everyone at Brown Books Publishing Group who helped make this book possible, including Milli Brown, Omar Mediano, Kathy Penny, Lucia Retta, Beth Robinson, and Danny Whitworth.

Chapter 1

It Starts Subtly Enough

"Why is there a hammer in the fridge?" I asked, surprised when I went to get a soda.

"Oh, that was just your father," my mother said. "He probably left it in there when he came inside to get some water." Mom credited my father's lack of attentiveness to the fact that he had been working in the sun too long. There seemed to be explanations for all of my dad's strange behaviors. He used to be very sharp, but recently he had started to forget little details. He would button his shirt the wrong way or put his morning slippers on backward and not notice. Or he'd ask questions when you had already given him an answer.

I was the first to notice something wrong with my dad, or at least the first to grow concerned about it. Everyone noticed the socket wrench in the lettuce drawer. But they blamed it on old age or stress.

"Oh, he just had a bad day . . . he's been smoking too much." He was still high functioning; he even worked as a handyman for my brother-in-law's painting company. He crafted many wooden projects in the shed in our backyard. My mother would insist that memory always tends to slip as people get older. I reasoned that she was probably right and stopped worrying about the little incidents. Then Dad lost his wallet.

It was clear that he was looking for it, but he wouldn't tell anyone that he had lost it. I saw him searching through all his pockets and every drawer. "Pop, are you looking for your wallet?"

"No, I'm not, China." China was my nickname.

"OK, because I saw where you left it. It's by the ashtray."

He ignored me and kept rummaging through the dresser. I walked away, but a few minutes later I saw him put his wallet in his pocket. Again, no big deal—my father had a very macho attitude. He couldn't let himself be shown up by a woman. But this kept happening. He left the wallet in the exact same spot every night, but he could never find it the following morning. It kept getting worse until it became "Somebody stole my wallet."

"Dad, there's only you, me, Mom, and Nora in the house, and Nora's too short to even reach the dresser. Who would have stolen your wallet?"

"I'm telling you somebody stole my wallet!" He was sure of it.

"It's exactly where you always leave it, by the ashtray."

"I know where I leave it, and it is not there. Someone broke in and stole it!"

"Really? Someone got past the security bars without breaking the windows, left the stereo and the TV, and just took your wallet—which is still by the ashtray."

"Exactly! We need to call the police!"

Finally, I picked it up and showed it to him. "Here! Your wallet is right here!" And like it was nothing, he took it and put it in his pocket.

It should be noted that my dad had been diagnosed with schizophrenia long before this started. He had been ill my entire life. Despite his affliction, he led a productive life. When he wasn't hospitalized, he worked as a draftsman. He designed and worked on some of the most important dams and monuments in Cuba. He was a great father and family man. During his good phases he made sure our family had everything we needed and then some. We were the only family on our block that had a refrigerator and a television. He planned ahead and saved up for the times when he would succumb to his mental illness and have to be hospitalized again. Watching my father's struggle and admiring his strength is what inspired me to become a psychiatrist.

Now I was starting to notice these little oddities in his behavior. All my training as a doctor told me these actions were not related to his primary mental illness. This was something different; all these quirks had to do with memory. He was forgetting his wallet, he was forgetting his tools, and he was forgetting what you had just told him two minutes ago. This was more than simple forgetfulness.

I knew Dad wasn't right, so I made it a point to touch base with his psychiatrist. The doctor, a pleasant and friendly man, told me there was nothing wrong with my father. "As you know," the doctor said, "he is ill—but he hasn't had any episodes for a while. I haven't noticed any changes in his condition. He's always very clear when he comes in. I like your dad. He always compliments me for being a good doctor; it's a real boost to the ego."

"That's Dad," I chuckled. Ever since the day I'd told him I was going to be a doctor, he had decreed all people of the medical field to be the best people in the world.

The doctor continued, "When he comes in, I ask how he's doing, if he is sleeping well, and he says that he is just fine and that he doesn't need the medication anymore."

"Well, that's nothing new." I added, "He always did that to his doctors in Cuba."

"Did what?"

"You know, flatter his doctors and try to convince them to take him off his medication. At every visit he would say things like, 'I don't need medication because I'm a man.'"

I noticed an odd expression on the doctor's face as he spoke. "You don't say."

I jumped forward in my seat, shocked at what I was starting to realize. "Do you mean to tell me that you've been taking him off his meds?"

"Oh, no, no, of course not . . . I've just cut down on his dosage."

My father had tricked his doctor. The doctor apologized for being duped. I was elated; I thought that I finally had an answer to my questions. This must have been the problem. Dad had been acting weird because the doctor had been tapering off his medications.

Something I've learned over the years is that in every diagnosis, you have to take into account the human factor. My dad lied to his doctors. People do that; they lie for various reasons. The doctor also assumed that my dad's schizophrenia was the cause of all his problems. I willingly accepted what the doctor told me even though I knew these symptoms were unrelated to schizophrenia; I reasoned that Dad's behavior was a reaction to his lack of medication. When Alzheimer's starts to manifest itself in a loved one, you try to explain the symptoms away; you look for an excuse for their strange behavior.

Dad resumed the correct dosage of his medication, but nothing really changed. There were still handsaws on the soda cans in the fridge. He was a little resentful that I had gone over his head and spoken to the doctor. The more I tried to correct him, the more he got upset with me. Now when I pointed out his wallet, he would glare at me, pull out his work journal, and scribble something down. I didn't know what he was writing, but I was sure it was some opinion of me that he didn't want me to hear. Nothing changed until he started having higher deficits.

I was home early one day when all of a sudden I heard my mother screaming.

"Trujillo, you burned the table!" I knew it had to be something bad because she was calling him by his last name. As I entered the living room, ready to play referee to one of my parents' old-married-couple squabbles, I saw my mother smothering the coffee table with the mop. "Look what you did!" she yelled at my father. "You and your stupid cigarettes! You could have burned the whole house down!"

When we looked at Dad, he was already lighting up another cigarette. "Woman, what are you talking about? This is my first one all day."

My mother grabbed the ashtray full of cigarette butts. "Then what do you call this?"

Dad scoffed at the ashtray. "That just shows how bad you are at cleaning. You should have cleaned that out last night."

Knowing my mother's obsession with keeping a clean house, I realized that this was a bold and dangerous accusation for my father to make. My mother's eyes blazed. She took a deep breath as if to fortify her lungs for the massive tongue lashing she was about to deliver. My five-year-old daughter, Nora, ran out of the room. She knew what was coming.

"Are you calling me sloppy? That's some nerve coming from a man who doesn't have the common sense to use an ashtray for the twentieth cigarette he smoked in one hour! No, you just think the coffee table is ugly, so you're just going to line up a row of lit cigarettes to see how many it takes to burn it to ash! But why stop at the table? Why not the whole house? Why not all of Florida? Don't expect me to vacuum up your charred carcass since I'm such a slob."

Dad didn't say a word. He just looked at her, pulled out his journal, wrote something down, closed the journal, and walked outside. Mom stayed glued to the spot, completely dumbfounded by Dad's lack of response. Then Nora came running out of the kitchen. She grabbed Dad's pack of cigarettes from the burnt coffee table and ran back to the kitchen.

"Nora, what are you doing?" I asked.

"Saving Florida!" she exclaimed as she dropped the pack into the garbage.

I knew Mom could be a bit melodramatic when she was upset, so I went out to the backyard to check on Dad. He was leaning against the wall of the house, smoking.

"Hey, China, did you just get home now?" *Oh my God!* I thought. *He forgot the whole argument, and he forgot I was there.*

I went back to the doctor because I could no longer justify Dad's symptoms. This was more than schizophrenia.

The doctor gave me more excuses. "Oh, he's aging. It's normal for people his age to start to forget things here and there."

I looked back at him and said, "He's not that old. He's only sixty. We don't have any family history of early onset dementia. This is more than just forgetting where he leaves his wallet. He's forgetting to put out his cigarettes. He leaves them anywhere and everywhere. It's becoming a hazard. He doesn't remember conversations moments after they take place." But the psychiatrist just brushed me off. So I took Dad to the medical doctor; they gave him a complete checkup and he was OK. But I still knew something was wrong.

When my father started to get Alzheimer's, people knew about the disease but nothing like they do today. They weren't familiar with its stages, and most people believed it was a normal part of growing old. This didn't matter much because there was no real treatment at the time. The only medications available were antipsychotics, which Dad was already taking. The medical doctor just told him to take vitamins. That didn't help.

When Dad was first diagnosed, I resolved to educate myself in the best way I could. I made use of my environment and observed patients in the psychiatric hospital where I worked. Patients of a certain age had a habit of becoming disoriented in the afternoon. This is now known as Sundowner Syndrome, and it's one of the three major symptoms of Alzheimer's. With sundown comes a decrease in stimuli. People with Sundowner Syndrome become disoriented, wander around, and do things that they would not do during the daytime. When my father got Alzheimer's, people didn't understand this symptom.

At the time, the nurses would say, "Oh, yeah, after three or four o'clock they begin to act worse. We give them their medication to put them to sleep so they won't disrupt the other patients." Watching those patients, I realized their symptoms matched my father's. I started to study everything I could about the condition. At the time, it was called Organic Brain Syndrome (OBS). Any elderly person who was a little confused, disoriented, or forgetful was referred to as OBS. It wasn't until the early nineties that Alzheimer's became common terminology.

Code Name: What's in a Name?

At the time my father started displaying symptoms of Alzheimer's, the doctors called it Organic Brain Syndrome. My mother would call it atherosclerosis, a Hispanic term that meant you were getting demented. My young daughter interpreted that as Arthur Sclerosis. Eventually we heard the word dementia—more specifically, "dementia of the Alzheimer's type." But I have yet to find a single person who liked any of those terms.

My own patients with Alzheimer's were very sensitive about the name. They would say, "I don't have Alzheimer's," or, "You're making that up." Of course, they were already in hospital care and had forgotten they had been diagnosed five years ago. Not so long ago, in some communities, any insinuation of dementia meant that the person had to be shipped away. Nobody wanted a crazy person in their family. You either sent them to an institution or locked them in the back room. Even in modern, civilized countries, mental illness still carries a stigma. So it can be very hard to say the word "Alzheimer's" around these patients.

So I found an alternative. Alzheimer's was discovered by a German doctor, Dr. Alois Alzheimer. The word for German in Spanish is *Aleman*. I started referring to the disease as the *Aleman*, or "the German." "Boy, the German is really acting up today," I would say to the nurses, or ask, "Did the German sleep last night?"

"Oh, no, Dr. T," they would reply (Dr. T is what most people call me). "That German was marching around from 2:00 to 6:00 a.m."

The best part was none of my Alzheimer's patients ever got upset over the term. In fact, some of them wanted to know who this misbehaving German was. Then an interesting thing happened. I was in the habit of talking to patients and their families about "the German." I started to notice that the family members were calmer when I used this code word. They found the term "German" less offensive than the word "patient." For all the qualities people generally associate with the word "German," illness isn't one of them. By no means is the use of this term meant to insult or offend anyone from Germany. Rather, it is in homage to the German doctors who discovered the disease, including German psychiatrist and neuropathologist Alois Alzheimer. In the medical field, it is a common practice to name a new discovery after someone who made great contributions to it. In keeping with this tradition, the nickname "German" for Alzheimer's patients is fitting.

If you're dealing with someone who is sensitive about his or her Alzheimer's (whether a patient or family member), it might be wise to come up with a code name. Of course, you do not have to use "German"—please feel free to use your own code. It sounds a little silly, but using a code name helps to disassociate your loved ones from their diagnoses, perhaps enough to allow them to process its reality. For example, it is less threatening to hear "Uncle Bobo did a dance today" than "Dad's Alzheimer's started acting up in the supermarket today." There are going to be plenty of times when you have to face serious issues with this disease. You should not take everything about it too seriously or too personally.

It's OK to make lighthearted remarks around Alzheimer's Dementia (AD) patients. The more outlandish the better; there's less chance that they will get upset unnecessarily. If every interaction with your loved one is a serious conversation about Alzheimer's, they will begin to sense a level of negativity. Even though it is not your intention to hurt the patient's feelings, that negativity will build upon itself and intensify. Eventually, it will become obvious even to someone who is losing their mind. When you associate negative feelings with the disease, you also associate them with the person. Even if you try to hide your frustration, it will show. This causes a rift between the patient and their family. If every reference to the disease is negative, any discussion you try to have about Alzheimer's is not going to be good. If you know conversations are not going to be pleasant, you start avoiding them. And if you associate the unpleasantness of Alzheimer's with the Alzheimer's patient, you start avoiding that person too.

However, an inside joke makes a conversation less grim, and people grow more comfortable discussing the problem. From now on, if you see the term German in this book, know that I am referring to someone with Alzheimer's. It's much easier than saying "your loved one with Alzheimer's" but maintains the same positive recognition of how much you care for the patient.

Once I knew (or thought I knew) what my family was dealing with when it came to my dad; I actually felt confident that I could handle it with no trouble at all.

I was wrong.

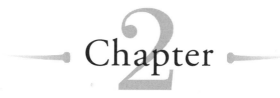

Alzheimer's History

S ince we've begun to discuss some of my own family's history with the disease, let's talk about the history of Alzheimer's. In fact, let's go ahead and get all the facts, stats, and data out of the way.

History

Alzheimer's disease was first identified in Germany by Emil Kraepelin and Aloysius "Alois" Alzheimer in the early twentieth century. The two psychiatrists worked at the Asylum for Lunatics and Epileptics (yes, that's the actual name translated into English). It was there that Dr. Alzheimer noticed a patient in her mid-fifties whose symptoms differed from standard "lunacy." She suffered from short-term memory loss, and her symptoms worsened as the sun set. Upon the patient's death, Alzheimer and Kraepelin examined her brain. With a newly developed technique, they used liquefied silver to chart the pathology in the histological section of the brain. The silver staining method allowed them to observe a buildup of amyloid plaques and neurofibrillary tangles in microscope slides.

When Alzheimer's was discovered in 1906, doctors did not fully understand the complexity of the disease. At the time, many accepted memory loss as a fact of life; it was generally expected that when you got older you would lose your memory or "go senile." As a result, doctors did not immediately identify Alzheimer's symptoms in the senior population. The first people diagnosed with Alzheimer's were in their forties or fifties and had what is now known as early-onset Alzheimer's. Of course, people do stand out if they're in their fifties and already developing senile dementia. Doctors later recognized the same symptoms in senior patients and began to diagnosis Alzheimer's within the elderly population. The growing number of cases led to expanded interest.

With the exception of early-onset Alzheimer's, there is no evidence to date that suggests Alzheimer's is a hereditary disease. In the past, cognitive tests were used to determine diagnosis, and these tests were only effective after dementia had already set in.

What is Alzheimer's Disease?

It may surprise you to learn that memory loss does not define Alzheimer's disease. Though a widely recognized symptom, memory loss is simply a by-product of the disease. Sound silly? Try to wrap your mind around it anyway. You need to understand this next time you get frustrated at your German because he doesn't remember where he left your car keys.

There is no straightforward definition of Alzheimer's disease (AD). Today, even the original, definitive findings of Alois Alzheimer are being questioned. I'm very sorry if that disappoints you. I can guarantee that it makes me equally frustrated and upset.

What I can tell you is this: Alzheimer's is a form of dementia. In fact, it is the most common form of presenile dementia. This means Alzheimer's disease is a psychiatric disorder. However, because most insurance companies don't provide psychiatric coverage (don't even get me started on this), Alzheimer's is classified as a condition of aging or primary care—which is why you will often hear doctors refer to it as "dementia of the Alzheimer's type."

Alzheimer's causes neurons in the brain to die. Dead neurons are replaced by senile (amyloid) plaques and neurofibrillary tangles. (Or it could be the other way around; we're no longer sure.) All Alzheimer's patients have a high concentration of neurofibrillary tangles and amyloid plaques in the temporal lobe. Now here's the twist in the tale: *most* old people have neurofibrillary tangles and amyloid plaques whether or not they have Alzheimer's. Heck, the human brain starts shrinking after age forty. The difference in Alzheimer's patients is the high concentration of plaques and tangles in certain areas of the brain, such as the temporal lobe.

Alzheimer's is a terminal disease, which means this disease will cause the brain to deteriorate until the person dies. Once the damage has been done, there is no going back. No treatment or procedure can repair damaged brain cells. Your best bet is to diagnose the disease early and slow down its symptoms.

I'm not going into the biochemical compound explanation of AD because, unless you're a doctor, you won't understand it. And if you are a doctor, you have your medical books for that. But I'll explain a few of the terms I will be using that the regular layperson might not understand.

- *Temporal Lobe*: The outer surface of the brain located in the temple regions. This area controls impulses. While the temporal lobe is highly affected by Alzheimer's, it is not the only area affected by the disease.
- *Neurons*: Brain cells. They relay messages between the brain and the body via chemical neurotransmitters.
- *Neurotransmitters*: The chemical agents that relay messages between neurons.
- *Amyloid Plaque*: Similar to the stuff the dentist scrapes off your teeth. It's a thick layer of proteins and cellular material that builds up and continues to grow as insoluble neurofibrillary tangles within the brain cells.
- *Neurofibrillary Tangles*: Twisted fibers that form inside brain cells and cause irreparable damage.

Diagnosis

Doctors will look for Alzheimer's by performing a series of simple tests, including

- **The Folstein Test, or mini-mental state examination (MMSE):** a simple question sheet.
- **Neuropsychological screening:** Doctors present the patient with a picture and ask them to reproduce it. Then they ask questions to test the patient's memory and comprehension.
- **Questioning the family or caretaker:** the most straightforward method of diagnosis. The patient might try to conceal his deficits, but a concerned family member or caretaker will report every symptom.

The PET scan, a more advanced technique, produces an electronic image of the brain that shows any loss of tissue due to senile plaque. Tissue damage also can be detected with a biopsy, but the risk of mortality as well as other complications, particularly for an older individual, makes a brain biopsy an unjustifiable diagnostic procedure. The only absolute way to positively identify Alzheimer's is to examine the brain in an autopsy.

Statistics

I'm only discussing statistics here because I know someone will want to see them. Let me point out now that 90 percent of these statistics will have an average of less than 1 percent of anything to do with you. Alzheimer's is personal. Yes, everyone will go through the same symptoms, and yes, it will affect the family; but everyone handles it differently. I know some of you have a tendency to freak out. You want to see numbers so you can calculate the risks or the chances or the probability. . . . Don't do that; it won't help.

The average life expectancy of a patient after he is diagnosed with AD is between four and ten years. However, my father lived for fifteen years after the initial onset of symptoms. There is no automatic shut-down clock that is activated when you get Alzheimer's.

An estimated twenty-six million people are affected by Alzheimer's, and that number is expected to quadruple by 2050. This number may be overwhelming, but remember that your task is to care for the one Alzheimer's patient whom you know. Not millions.

More than half of the people currently residing in nursing homes have Alzheimer's. A very good reason to be considerate to the staff if your one person ends up in a facility that may be dealing with twenty similar cases. Keep in mind that most stays in nursing homes are temporary; most patients don't live there full time.

The ε4 allele gene is present in 50 percent of Alzheimer's patients. In statistical talk, 50 percent means a chance of yes and a chance of no. So a German either will have the gene or he won't. It is still being debated whether this gene (or four hundred others) is connected to AD.

Alzheimer's affects 5 percent of people over the age of sixty-five, and the chances of getting it increase with every year—up to 15 to 25 percent for people over the age of eighty-five. AD mostly affects people who are sixty-five or older (with the rare exception of early-onset Alzheimer's). The same goes for osteoporosis, loss of hearing, loss of vision, tiredness, hatred for the loud music teenagers are listening to, incontinence, inability to process dairy products, erectile dysfunction, getting store discounts on Tuesdays . . . you see where this is going. AD doesn't run on a schedule. My father got it early in his sixties. You are not going to get AD the moment you blow out the candles on your sixty-fifth birthday cake. And you don't have to finish out each year saying, "Woo, I managed to dodge the bullet this time." At a certain age, your body is going down no matter what, so if you don't have any responsibilities pending, just do whatever you want to do now.

Increased Risk Factors

I have the same hesitation here as I did with the statistics. Someone out there is going to look at this, calculate their own possibilities of getting Alzheimer's, and start worrying. So I want to emphasize: to date, scientists do not know what triggers Alzheimer's. These risk factors are, at best, scientific shots in the dark.

I'm just going to say this: no one knows for certain who will develop Alzheimer's. Very few people can predict when someone will get sick. Those who can are usually found in creepy sci-fi movies. If you don't know for sure whether someone is going to get Alzheimer's, how can you say that they did or didn't because of certain factors? If you don't know when someone is going to die, how can you say definitively that x, y, or z shortened their life span? Keep this is mind when you hear anyone start saying, "This will lower your chances," or, "This will increase the risk."

Increased risk factors for developing AD include being a woman, having Down syndrome, having other diseases of the brain like Huntington's or Parkinson's, an unbalanced diet, writing with a simple handwriting style, head injury, limited social interactions, and hereditary factors. So where do we start?

Unbalanced Diet

Well, that gets blamed for everything. Let me skip to the end and let you know that there is *no* solid proof linking junk food to AD.

Diseases of the Brain

I find this one especially interesting because my father did have a preexisting mental illness. For more on this, please see the section on studies and theories later in this chapter.

Head Injury

Trauma to the head can cause a number of mental changes, especially if it caused damage to the brain. But not everyone with AD has suffered a head injury, and not everyone who has been bumped on the head develops AD. You might be looking at a case in which an older person falls down and later gets diagnosed with Alzheimer's. It is more than likely that the fall did not cause AD but that AD caused the fall. Loss of coordination is a symptom of Alzheimer's; that's why AD patients often fall.

Being a Woman

Sorry, but this is true. Women are twice as likely to develop Alzheimer's disease. But consider the fact that there are generally more women in the elderly population than men. In the sixty-five and older range, the male population really decreases. There is an average of eighty-three men per every hundred women between the ages of sixty-five and seventy-five. You're also more likely to have a nana than a papaw at ninety; for the ages of eighty-five and over there are only forty-six grandpas per hundred grandmas. Women have a tendency to live longer than men by an average of about five years. So one could argue that more women develop AD because women live longer. Having breasts does not guarantee that you will get AD the minute you turn sixty-five. But some scientific studies suggest a genetic reason that women are more susceptible. For more information on those studies, see the section on studies and theories.

Limited Social Interactions

I can understand the theory that someone who is all alone with no friends or family would start to deteriorate mentally. But if you are reading this now, you probably care for someone who got sick. Your loved one had support and got sick anyway. Even presidents—who have to interact with all these other countries, a skill that requires great thinking capacity—have suffered from AD. Know this now: you did not fail your loved one. They did not get sick because you didn't spend enough time with them. They were already going to get sick. Now you just have to focus on treating them.

Hereditary Factors

Approximately 10 percent of patients who suffer from Alzheimer's have a family history of the disease. That means about 90 percent have no relatives who were similarly affected. There is no solid proof to date that confirms AD as a hereditary disease.

Handwriting

I'm not making this up. Someone really did a study and found that a percentage of his subjects with AD had a very simple handwriting style when they were younger. I'm sorry, but if there were a real connection between simple handwriting and AD, then no doctor would ever get Alzheimer's.

Possible Preventatives

These are the opposite of the risk factors. Below, we'll discuss some behaviors that supposedly reduce your chances of developing AD. Remember, doing one or all of these things doesn't mean you are safe from developing Alzheimer's. So if there is no guarantee that these activities will prevent AD, why bother? Because these activities *have* been proven to stimulate the brain and activate neurons. Furthermore, these activities will reduce the effects of other mental deficiencies. That's why we have arts and crafts in the psychiatric ward.

At a certain age, everything in the human body starts going downhill. As I mentioned before, the brain usually starts to shrink around age forty. Often this is very minor with minimal effect, but everyone will experience some loss of mental capacity in one form or another. So if these activities do help to shore up your brain against mental decline *and* there is a chance they can prevent AD, what have you got to lose?

The preventatives, in no particular order, are chess, crossword puzzles, Sudoku, reading, writing, socializing, board games, riddles, jigsaw puzzles, speaking a second language, learning a new language, and, in fact, all learning in general. The list goes on, but here's the short version: anything that involves learning or requires you to use your comprehension and problem-solving skills is good exercise for your brain.

Now daily activities alone don't really cut it. Why? Because if you're a master chef, cooking is a routine for you. You already know what to do, and you're functioning on previously held knowledge. The same thing goes for a hobby, whether it's tinkering with cars or wood crafts. This doesn't mean you should stop your favorite craft. Quite the contrary: it's a call to take on new, more complicated projects. You know the ones—the ones that make you think, *Wow, that is so cool, but I could never do anything like that. I don't have the skill or know the technique.* Now you officially have a medical excuse to try it out. You don't know how? Learn. The guys who did it first had to start somewhere too. Study their techniques. The more difficult the activity is, the better for your brain and the greater the feeling of accomplishment you will have when you finish.

But what if you're not a cook or a craftsman? What if you're a sports fan? I guarantee you that, as much as you may know about sports, there is always more to learn. Read up on the history of the game or the players. Study their techniques and strategies. "Honey, I have to call Mike over to discuss the pros and cons of a pinch hitter. It's important for my mental health. It might keep you from having to put me in a nursing home one day." Who could object to that?

Studies and Theories

When my father first got sick, there were very few studies being conducted on Alzheimer's. Now there are more than five hundred studies in progress. Keep a sharp eye out for articles that report, "A new study *suggests* . . ." This means they're still theorizing and the results are not conclusive. Remember that researchers are under a lot of pressure. Often they've received a grant from people who want to see results. To avoid losing their funding, they publish the first results they have even if they're not definitive. Also keep in mind when reading recent studies that some may be insufficiently funded or may not have a broad range of test subjects. Some conduct research in very small groups, and the results really only apply to that group. (For example, the study that suggests simple handwriting is an increased risk factor was done in an isolated community.) One day these studies may make a breakthrough, but my point is that you shouldn't worry yourself too much over things you read.

Some experiments include factors that you would probably never associate with disorders of the brain. For example, recent studies have examined shark tissue and cobra venom. Don't laugh—for all you know a snake bite may end up curing

Alzheimer's! And I'm not going to sit here and discredit the methods of any scientist because you'd be surprised how many scientific breakthroughs have been discovered through unconventional methods or even by accident. Plus, new studies published two years down the line probably will discredit today's findings. There's always something new to uncover.

Theories

Extended Life Span

According to this theory, Alzheimer's is simply a natural risk of aging. Given better medical knowledge and living conditions, the life expectancy of humans has increased substantially since the Industrial Revolution. Once the life expectancy of the average man was about forty years. That's nearly doubled today. Some scientists believe the human body was not meant to live so long and that, as a result, the body just starts to fall apart.

Down Syndrome

Before 1980, the life expectancy for someone with Down syndrome was around twenty-five years. Today, with the help of more advanced drugs, that average has risen to sixty years. Interestingly enough, almost everyone with Down syndrome who lives to age fifty develops Alzheimer's. (In people with Down syndrome, Alzheimer's usually sets in between the ages of forty and fifty.) Many researchers believe that the mutation of the twenty-first chromosome, the most common genetic cause of Down syndrome, may explain the Alzheimer's-like symptoms that Down syndrome patients experience. The question remains: is this comorbidity related to the theory of extended life expectancy, or do Down syndrome patients develop Alzheimer's because of a preexisting deficit in the brain? We simply don't know yet.

Genetics

I know I'm going to step on someone's ego here. Geneticists have proposed many theories as to which gene is responsible for Alzheimer's. As mentioned above, there is a study investigating whether the ε4 allele gene associated with Down syndrome may be connected to AD. Essentially, AD may be triggered by the same defective genes that lead to other mental disorders. The list of suspects is currently around four hundred genes.

Geneticists search for an explanation in genetics because that's what they study. Those who study infectious disease would look for a virus; an oncologist would look for a tumor; each is drawn to search for a cause within their field. That's why oncological research finds cancer-causing material in orange juice. Don't get me wrong, I'm not insulting geneticists or their research. Genetic research has advanced medicine greatly. No, the problem is you. Yes, you! When you hear the term *genetics*, you assume the facts are predetermined and set in stone. But let me clarify what geneticists are doing in their study of Alzheimer's: they are doing *research* into the *theory* that there is a genetic factor to the disease. And as of yet they have no solid conclusions; everything is still theory. Two years from now, many of these theories may be obsolete. Geneticists may even find that there is no hereditary element to Alzheimer's. So, you, calm down. Genetic research is difficult enough as it is without you adding to the sensationalism.

Estrogen

As I mentioned already, more women are affected by Alzheimer's than men. There is still a debate as to whether the disease is associated with the X chromosome or with any other genes whose incidence is higher in women. However, studies involving estrogen hormone replacement in menopausal women seem to demonstrate that estrogen can reduce the likelihood of developing AD. Scientists believe that estrogen helps keep neurons alive.

Diabetes

According to this theory, those who have diabetes are less likely to have Alzheimer's (or advanced Alzheimer's). By no means am I recommending that you should attempt to develop diabetes on purpose to avoid getting Alzheimer's.

Preexisting Condition

This theory indicates that people with preexisting mental conditions are more likely to develop Alzheimer's. Such conditions include Parkinson's, Huntington's, schizophrenia, and Down syndrome. The theory postulates that these cognitive differences leave the door open for Alzheimer's.

Antipsychotic Drugs

A new study suggests that the antipsychotics used to treat Alzheimer's increase the patient's chances of dying sooner. But as I mentioned in the sections on preventatives and risk factors, if you're not sure when someone is going to die, how can you say their life span has been shortened? That doesn't mean the theory must be wrong; it might turn out to be 100 percent right. But then what? Should you take the medicines that offer a better quality of life at the cost of a shorter life span, or vice versa? That's a decision you would have to make on your own.

At this time, the prevailing theory is that AD is triggered by a combination of genetic (whether hereditary or mutated) and acquired damage to brain cells along with the naturally occurring deterioration of brain cells that comes with age.

Chapter 3

The First Big Incident

Wandering is one of the "Big Three" symptoms of Alzheimer's, along with memory loss and sundowning. For these reasons, Alzheimer's patients require constant monitoring.

To gain some insight, consider this: You've probably walked into a room and then forgotten why you went in there. In this situation, you likely retraced your steps and tried to remember what you were doing. When Alzheimer's patients experience the same thing, however, they don't think to go back. They'll start off looking for something, but when they forget what it is, they just keep going. They won't stop until something or someone else catches their attention. The Alzheimer's mind doesn't process what happened two minutes ago; it only focuses on what's immediately in front of it. It can remember twenty years ago, but not the last two minutes.

Dealing with Conflict

The number one rule when dealing with Alzheimer's patients is to avoid conflict. But there *will* be conflicts, whether they arise with outside sources, with family members, or with the Germans themselves. And because Alzheimer's patients, unaware of their limitations, often cause problems, caretakers naturally may develop a feeling of resentment directed toward them. One time when my father wandered off, I had to deal with the cops, an angry mob, upset patients who didn't appreciate having to wait for me to get back to work, coworkers who didn't like dealing with the upset patients, and a boss who didn't like the fact that everyone else was upset! In just one incident, at least forty people were upset with me.

I easily could have blamed my dad for the whole disaster. But it wasn't his fault. He was sick; he didn't know what he was doing. I could have blamed my mom for not keeping a better eye on him except that it was all new to her too. Dad had been acting fine before. How was she to know he was about to start wandering? And if I were to pin the blame on my mother, she could turn right around and pin it on me. Why couldn't I do more to help? I was working . . . but you see where this is going.

Most of the emotional trauma associated with Alzheimer's stems from such conflicts. These situations will cause you to feel frustrated, embarrassed, or angry. It's almost a reflex to take out these negative emotions on someone else. Even people who manage to hide their emotions under a cool façade will end up with a stockpile of resentment and anger that will eventually explode at the wrong moment.

First off, get away from the blame game. Remind yourself that the real culprit is a disease, not a person. Blaming other family members only creates more anger—and you'll inevitably start to associate that anger with the German. When your loved one is first diagnosed with Alzheimer's, it's a new and confusing situation for everyone. Most people won't see an Alzheimer's patient; they'll continue to see the family member they've always known having a few odd moments. They'll be overconfident in the individual's ability to function normally. People will get distracted, guards will be dropped, and mistakes will be made.

When that happens, don't start pointing fingers. You want the whole family in this together. When a mistake occurs, bring the whole family together without anger or blame. Sit everyone down and discuss. "This is the problem; how can we fix it? How can we prevent it from happening again?" Get everyone's input. As a family, figure out a routine in which the German will be supervised constantly. Alzheimer's can put a great deal of stress on a family. But if you can handle your own stress and push the anger aside, an Alzheimer's diagnosis can bring a family closer together.

If a confrontation arises between your German and someone outside the family, try to explain: "Please understand, my father is sick. He has Alzheimer's and doesn't know what he's doing." Avoid saying "I'm sorry" if you can. Some people out there interpret that as an admission of liability—which could invite a lawsuit! Ask for understanding, not forgiveness.

Wandering

I remember the first time I realized I was in over my head. That day I was working in the emergency room when I got a call from my mother, who screamed, "I'm trapped in a golden cage!"

"What? Mom, you're not making any sense."

"Your father left to put an envelope in the mailbox. An empty envelope! He locked all the doors and took all the keys with him."

Back then the neighborhood was a bit iffy, so I had installed security bars on all of the windows and doors. Security bars can be opened only with a key. My mother told me that Dad had been working in the yard. He had taken a set of keys with him and forgot to put them back on the key hook when he came inside. When he went into the kitchen, he saw the mail that had just arrived. In his mind, mail equaled mailbox. He reasoned that this envelope had to be mailed (he didn't notice that it was an incoming letter and had already been opened). He picked it up, told my mother he was going to the mailbox, took the second and last set of keys, and walked out the front door. As he did this, my mother started to wonder what envelope he was talking about. Then she looked out the window and saw him walking off in the wrong direction. She went to the front door to call him back only to realize it was locked. The one thing Dad did remember was to lock the security door to keep his family safe.

"Then what's the problem, Ma? Just wait for him to get back."

"He left two hours ago!"

"What? And you waited till now to call me?"

I had to drop everything in the middle of the day, get another doctor to cover me in the psychiatric ER, and drive from Jackson Memorial Hospital to my house, which was over twenty-five miles away. I didn't have to think about everything that could go wrong because I had just gotten a brand-new cell phone, which my mother kept calling every five minutes to relate possible scenarios. "He must have been hit by a car . . . He could have walked into gang territory . . . He's probably been assaulted . . . The drug dealers must have kidnapped him . . . What's taking you so long? If the house catches fire, your daughter and I will both die a horrific death."

I finally got home and unlocked the security door. The first thing my daughter did was to jump in the car and say, "I'll help you find Grandpa." I think she wanted to escape the "horrible death" that her grandmother had been describing for the last hour. We drove down the street in the direction my mother had seen him go. I spotted him just as we reached 103rd Street, still holding the envelope. I drove about half a block ahead of him and parked the car. When he saw me coming down the sidewalk toward him, he said, "Finally, I've been waiting for you. Here, you have to put this in the mailbox."

To avoid a similar disaster, I made about twenty copies of the security keys and gave them to all our neighbors. If Dad ever locked my mother in the house again, it would be easier for her to call one of them rather than waiting for me to drive all the way home from the hospital. But from that point on, the security bars were completely useless because anyone who wanted to get into the house could just use the key.

The supervision system we had in place wasn't working. Mom would allow Dad to pretty much continue his normal routine. Then she would be surprised when he wandered away. Then I would drive home from work to find him. I started thinking of what I could do differently.

That night, I wrote all of my phone numbers on a card and showed it to Dad. I explained that if he were lost, he could use it to call me. To make sure he knew how to use it, I wrote on the top of the card: *Dad, if you are lost, call Moraima at this number.* I figured that even if he forgot why he had the card, he could read the instructions.

His response was typical: "I'm never going to need that. I never get lost. Why are you giving this to me?"

I knew that if I reminded him that he did get lost, it would only upset him more—and he'd write who knows what about me in his journal. I managed to convince him I was doing this "because of my new cellular phone. It's a new number,

Dad, and I want you to keep it in your wallet if you need to call me."

"Oh, OK," he said. He put it in his wallet.

Wait, I remembered, *he forgets where he leaves the wallet every morning.* So I made another card and put it in his pants pocket; he definitely never forgot his pants. But he did change his mind about which pants he wanted to wear. So I made more copies, enough for every pocket of every article of clothing he owned.

Of course he would have been insulted if I'd said, "Hey, let's put all these emergency cards in your pants so that if you ever get lost again you'll know how to call." I knew his response would have been the same as before: "I never get lost. You are treating me like a child. How dare you be so disrespectful to your father?" Or he probably would have put all the cards in one pocket, which was no good.

Instead of having to deal with that, my mother and I sneaked into Dad's room while he was taking a shower. As my mother helped me put the emergency contact cards in all those pockets, she was struck by a thought.

"Won't all these papers bleed and fall apart when I do the laundry?" *Oh.* Of course, her only concern was that this would stain the clothes, but she still had a point. The next opportunity I had, I took everything Dad ever wore, even his underwear, and wrote on the tags in permanent marker. I wrote, *If found, call* . . . followed by my cell number and beeper.

Imagine my surprise the first time I got a call.

"Is this Mrs. Mori . . . Mo-ram-mi Tru-jill . . . Tru-jello?"

"Yes, this is *Dr. Trujillo*. And whom am I speaking with?" I asked, a little miffed at this man who butchered my name.

"This is Sergeant Kolsky with the Hialeah Police Department. We've found your father." *Oh my God. Found him? I didn't even know he was lost!* The police officer continued, "He's at McDonald Park. We found your number in his wallet."

"What happened? Is he all right?"

"Ah, yeah, yeah. Some very . . . concerned mothers called us. Would you like to pick him up yourself, or do you want us to take him to a hospital?"

"No! Thank you, Mr. Officer, sir! I'll be right over!"

I raced to the park. When I arrived, I saw what can best be described as a mob trying to get to my father as the police put him in the back of their car. I ran up. "Wait, stop, you don't have to do that! He's harmless."

The police officer told me, "I know that, miss, but we have to do this to calm down the crowd. But I've been out here. I've been watching. He was just playing around with the kids; there was absolutely nothing perverse about any of his actions. Your father was taking the kids, helping them on the swings, putting them on the slides."

"Then if you know that, why are putting him in a patrol car?"

"Ma'am, please let me explain. He was also cleaning the sand off their butts when they fell down. This would upset any mother, but it's worse now because there was a child abducted at the mall recently."

All this time, the group of women continued to express their outrage. "Yeah, take him away!" "Lock him up!" "Take that dirty old man and throw him in jail." They were yelling all these horrible things that I knew were not true.

I said to the officer, "Look, give me a chance to talk to them and I'm sure—"

"I wouldn't do that if I were you, ma'am. We're the police and we just barely have them under control now. Just let us put him in the car till they leave."

I reasoned that he was right, so I said to go ahead. Not that they waited for my permission. I fretted and worried about how this would affect Dad. When the crowd finally dispersed I went to get him from the patrol car.

He was smiling. "China, did you see that? The police let me ride in their car. This makes me a very important person."

I asked him, "Dad, what were you doing?"

"I was playing with the grandkids. Then this gang showed up, but I was there to protect the children. Luckily the police came to assist me—which was good because those people were crazy."

As much as I had worked with police and the mentally ill, this was still a very difficult situation. Feelings of frustration and inadequacy overwhelmed me. Those parents believed my dad was trying to harm their children—and I had no way to convince them otherwise.

The Best Medicine

Even in difficult and painful situations, you simply cannot allow the negative emotions to get the best of you. Just let them go.

I know—it's easier said than done. I've dealt with people who tell me, "All I need to do is count to ten and the anger just melts away." Yet even as they speak, I notice that their fists are clenched. So what is the best way to avoid getting upset about these incidents?

Laugh. Of course you're going to be upset when you can't find your German and end up getting a call from the cops. But afterward, when you look back, you can generally find something to laugh about. When I got back to work that particular day and all my colleagues were upset, I started telling the story. "Leave it to my dad to single-handedly start a riot. There he is, 'defending the grandkids' from this crazed gang of housewives. And then, when the police show up, Dad thinks he is a VIP." They laughed. You can laugh at it!

Chapter 4

Memory Loss

Memory loss, the hallmark symptom of Alzheimer's, occurs when neurofibrillary tangles replace dead brain cells. As it loses capacity and memory, the brain attempts to compensate by reaching for any kind of stimulation in order to keep functioning. However, the tangles sometimes prevent the brain from remembering new experiences. Therefore, the brain either will search for stimuli in the long-term memory or look to something more concrete, like whatever is directly in front of it at the time. The park incident exemplifies this scenario. My father's mind lapsed and he started wandering until he found himself at the park. There he saw the children playing. His brain focused all of his immediate attention on these children. Then Dad fell back on his long-term memory to explain who they were and what he was doing there. He had memories of grandchildren, so his brain told him that the children in front of him were his grandchildren. The angry mothers who said otherwise were wrong. He simply lacked the short-term memory function he needed to fully comprehend the situation.

In the park, my father's behavior upset a number of outsiders, but most of the time the person who gets angry and frustrated is the caretaker. Say you are taking care of your dad, whose memory is not that good. For a brief moment he is totally, absolutely, positively convinced that he did something—even though you're telling him that he didn't. You're going to get into an endless argument that may even have a violent outcome, and you're not going to get anywhere. Your best bet is to stop pressing the point.

You shouldn't get upset over mistakes because everyone makes them, especially in the beginning. Dad functioned so well that at times I even forgot he was sick, which was a big mistake. But since I was a single, working mom, it was hard to take care of everything by myself. I took any help I could get.

"Dad, I have to help Nora with her homework. Do you think you can fix her bath so that when she's done I can just drop her in?"

"No problem, China," he said.

It was late and I was helping my daughter with her first report project. After we finished that, there was the rest of her homework, the extra math exercises we gave her, and her half hour of reading practice. This took a little longer than I anticipated, but we finally finished. I got up from the table and *splash*. I was standing in a stream of water. Where was it coming from? Nora shouted, "Puddles!" and tried to jump in them. I grabbed her before she could start splashing around and make a bigger mess. Carrying Nora so she didn't get wet, I followed this miniature river to the overflowing bathtub. My house was flooded. And where was Dad?

I finally found him smoking in the backyard. "Dad, why didn't you turn the water off?"

"What?"

"You left the water running."

"No, I didn't."

"Yes, after I asked you to prepare Nora's bath."

"No, you didn't."

"Dad, the house is flooded."

"No, it isn't."

He was actually standing next to a puddle where the water had leaked out the back door. I figured there was no point in arguing because I just wanted to clean up the place. "OK, fine, but you still have to help me mop all this up."

He just gave me a cheeky look, lit another cigarette, and said, "No, I don't."

Even things that seem very simple can snowball very quickly. I understand you're busy, you're in a rush. The only person available is your dad. It's only some minor task; he should have no problem with it. Are you a betting person? It might be something simple, something he was once capable of doing very easily, but now he has Alzheimer's. There's a chance, especially if it's late in the day, that he'll get halfway through the task and forget what he's doing. Even if you can get away with such assignments for a while, there is always the probability that something will go wrong.

One could argue that because Dad was still in the early stages, I could have avoided the whole situation by giving him more concrete instructions: Fill the tub for Nora's bath. When the tub is full, turn the water off and let me know. Nora argued that the flood could have been avoided if we hadn't given her so much homework. Of course, it might not always be homework. It could be something else—a quick run to the supermarket for milk, a phone call, the season finale of your favorite show that you just can't miss. There are always distractions.

But then I made another mistake. I tried to make him see the mistake he had made. Conflict will arise when you confront an Alzheimer's patient and try to make yourself heard instead of listening. You try to make the patient see the mess he has made; you try to make him remember your name. You don't listen when he says he doesn't. Remember, the most important thing is to avoid conflict. Don't try to win because that's how you will lose.

One time I got home early and made dinner for the family. We sat down at the dinner table together. Dad always had what some would call a pretty healthy appetite. To this day I'm surprised that he never just picked up the plate and swallowed it whole. On this occasion (just like at every other meal) he finished before the rest of us. He looked around the table, turned to my mom, and said, "Woman, where is my food?"

"You just finished eating it," she told him.

My father responded, "I'm not kidding, where is my food? You served everybody else and not your husband!"

Of course, his plate was sitting right there in front of him, but it was empty and everyone else at the table was eating. His mental process probably went something like this: "People eating . . . meal time . . . I should be eating . . . I am not eating . . . I have not been served!'

"There is no way you're still hungry!" my mother said.

"Of course I'm hungry, I haven't eaten!"

"You just finished eating."

"No, I didn't."

At this point I was holding my head. By now I'd learned to avoid conflict, but my mother didn't buy into that. According to her: One, my dad wasn't really sick. Two, she was his wife, which made her exempt from the "Don't confront Dad" rule. And three, if I told her otherwise, I would end up in a conflict with her!

Meanwhile, Nora was laughing. And she was right; to someone on the outside, the situation was hilarious. My father was oblivious; my mother was growing more and more frustrated trying to win the argument; and I couldn't make either one of them stop. It was like we were living in a sitcom. Nora thought Grandpa was playing a prank. We had done similar things with her and her cousins. The problem was the more she laughed, the angrier my mother got.

Finally I got up and said, "Here, just give him a little more food."

Of course, when he saw that he was given just a little bit more, he said, "You think I'm a fool? You don't want to feed me anymore. Am I not the man of this house?" And he went on and on until I finally figured it out.

"OK, Mom, from now on just serve him half of his food. Leave the other half in the microwave. If he pulls this stunt again, you can pull the other plate out of the microwave." She looked at me as if I were the one with dementia.

"Yeah, and what if he forgets he ate after the second plate, what am I supposed to do then? Cook him another meal and keep feeding him until he dies from his stomach exploding like a frog?" She had a very good point. But at least with my approach, we managed to pacify him for a little bit longer whenever he grew forgetful during a meal.

Most people assume that Alzheimer's patients act strange because they are losing their intelligence along with their memory. On the contrary, to compensate for short-term memory loss, the brain becomes ultra alert. It forgets what happened two minutes ago, but when it sees the empty plate it responds automatically. Because our Germans' brains are constantly on alert, their perception of events is very easily influenced by stimuli in their environment.

From the park experience I learned to predict which things will grab the German's attention. My father probably didn't plan to go to the park that day. He was wandering down the street and saw children playing. He loved my daughter Nora and her cousins so much that they were constantly in his thoughts—even when he couldn't recognize them. As a result, he associated all small children with his grandchildren. That's why he found himself drawn to the park when he saw the children playing there.

Think of things that grab the attention of your German. Is he always thinking of food? Does she have a thing for fancy cars? Sometimes Alzheimer's patients keep ending up in the same places after each memory lapse. When our loved ones wander off, it is very important to think like they do.

Bounty Hunter

The next time it wasn't the police who called but my mother. I was in the middle of a meeting at work. I had to excuse myself, find someone to cover for me, and take off. As I sped toward my house, I asked my mother where she had last seen Dad. "He was in the backyard."

If he had exited through the gate in the backyard, he would have kept going down the street. I immediately thought, *He's going back to the park.* I drove down to the park, but there was no sign of him. The park was empty. This was bad. Now I had no idea where he could have gone.

Relax, I told myself, *take a deep breath.* Then I tried to put myself in his frame of mind. *I'm walking down the street going to the park . . . wait! There are no kids in the park.* He didn't stop there because he didn't see any grandkids to play with. He would be wandering around still. From the park corner he could have gone three different ways. Something told me he wouldn't have gone straight ahead because the avenue was too crowded. He would have stayed on the larger roads, the main streets. I had a hunch that he turned right.

I drove up the street, scanning everyone on the sidewalk. Block after block, I drove and found nothing. I stopped just short of the expressway. He wouldn't have gone on the expressway. All the fast-moving cars would have scared him back. But by now he could have walked up to the expressway and turned around or just as easily gone down another street. I made a U-turn and drove more slowly. There had to be something I had missed.

This time I didn't just look at the people. I scanned everything that could have caught his attention. The street had plenty of little cafés that sold the Cuban coffee he loved so much. There were also several little markets; he could have gone inside to buy cigarettes. But of course he had left his wallet at home, so he didn't have any money. If he had tried to buy anything with no money on him, I figured the police would have called me by now, or at least there would have been some kind of commotion outside the establishment. But what else could have called his attention? As I looked to the left, I noticed an American flag waving majestically in the sky.

Even before he left his native country of Cuba, my father had a very patriotic devotion to the United States. His obsession with the American flag even featured in his schizophrenic psychosis. If he had seen a flag that large, he would have headed toward it. I made a left at the traffic light and drove toward the flag, which stood in the middle of a large shopping center.

As I drove into the plaza I noticed two women rushing out of the Toys"R"Us. I was sure he had followed the flag to the shopping center, and then noticed small children going in to shop. I parked and poked my head into the store. Inside, I heard a woman screaming. Found him!

I followed the sound of screaming down an aisle, and sure enough, there was Dad. He held a bunch of toys in one arm and was trying to hide a toddler behind his back to protect the child from a crazed, screaming woman. As store employees gathered around, my dad saw me coming and said, "Oh, there you are. Go ahead and pay him."

Pay . . . pay who? Pay for what?

"I told him you were a doctor."

Oh, Dad, whatever I'm going to pay just got doubled.

The store manager said, "Miss, your father has been here for some time. He says he's been shopping with his grandkids."

"I was shopping with the kids." By kids, he meant my daughter, niece, and nephews. But the toddler whose hand he was holding wasn't one of them. In his mind, the idea of kids went with the idea of a toy store. Since his grandkids weren't there when he arrived, he probably decided to buy them presents. For the last hour he'd been walking up and down this store, cramming toys into his arms and looking for "grandkids." He walked up to a little boy and handed him some toys. At first, the boy's grandmother was very flattered at this cute gesture. Of course, hers was the most adorable little boy in the world; who wouldn't stop to praise him? And take his little hand and walk off with him. . . . Wait. What?

Apparently that last part unnerved the boy's grandmother.

I was grateful that I had managed to find Dad before things got out of hand. This time, everyone was very understanding; the shoppers and employees figured out that Dad was mentally ill. I didn't even have to pay for anything. On the way home, after I got Dad in the car, I couldn't help thinking I was a little bit like Sherlock Holmes. The thought brought a smile to my face. I had tracked down Dad. "Elementary, my dear Watson." I got home and explained what happened to everyone in the house. My pride was crushed when my daughter looked at me and all she wanted to know was, "Where's my present?"

Chapter 5

Learning to Speak Alzheimer's

How do you talk to someone who doesn't recognize you? Communicating with an Alzheimer's patient is very frustrating, and it can be emotionally draining if you let it. Don't start getting sad over the situation because otherwise you will never be able to look your German in the face again. It's just another trial in your life; you've survived a couple. This is how you deal with it: You're going to learn to speak Alzheimer's.

Speaking Alzheimer's is like talking to a small child. If you've had one or have seen people with babies, you know about baby talk. Parents use very simple words. Apply the same rule to the German. Don't complicate sentences with long statements and lots of details. Alzheimer's patients are back at a very basic level, and if you say, "Mom, do you know who I am?" they're going to stare at you blankly. How does a baby learn to match his mother's name with her face? Every time the baby sees his mother, her face says "Mama." So he repeats the word "Mama" and that face smiles back at him. Unlike babies, Alzheimer's patients have a large vocabulary, but they have lost the capacity to use it. So keep it simple. Here are some guidelines that have helped me to communicate more effectively with my dad.

- **Have patience.** Remember that it will be tested.
- **Always approach from the front.** If you sneak up behind your German, you'll find out what happens, but don't say I didn't warn you.
- **Listen.** The best way to communicate with a German is to listen. Show that you're listening and trying to understand; encourage him to express himself even if he is having difficulties.
- **Maintain eye contact.** This is simple, but it shows you're listening. You can also get his attention by simply touching him and guiding him to look at you.
- **Be friendly.** Stay calm with a gentle expression, even if you really just want to hit him over the head with a frying pan. Don't let frustration get the best of you.
- **Don't criticize.** If he's stumbling around, don't call him out on it. It doesn't matter if he says something wrong; it doesn't even matter if he's making sense. If he says one thing and you say the opposite, you're creating a conflict.

- **Avoid conflict.**
- **Don't lose your patience and interrupt.** Offer assistance as necessary but know when to back off.
- **Avoid drilling or quizzing.** Don't ask questions like, "Don't you know who I am?" If he doesn't, asking can't make him remember and will only aggravate him.
- **Keep things short and sweet.** Speak slowly and clearly using simple words, especially when you are giving instructions.
- **Ask one question at a time and give him time to answer.** Don't run questions together: "Hi, Dad, how are you feeling today? Is everything good?" That's two questions.
- **Stick to safe subjects.** Try to avoid talking about anything that will upset him.
- **Address him by name and identify yourself.** "Hi Dad, it's me, your daughter, Moraima." You don't have to say your last name. He knows his last name.
- **Use pointing and touching to identify.** If I were to say, "Look, your granddaughter, Nora, came with me," my dad might not put two and two together. But if I put my hand around Nora while I say it, he might start to comprehend.
- **Don't talk about him as if he's not in the room.** He might have Alzheimer's, but he's still aware of what you're saying about him, and he's likely to take your attitude as criticism.

Let me give you an example of effectively greeting someone with Alzheimer's.

"Hey Mom, I'm John, your son. I'm here to see you." And guess what's going to happen: that face is going to smile.

"John, my son."

Chances are that if she repeats your name she might be able to recognize you. The proof that she does: for the rest of that visit she will repeat "John" when she talks to you and may even remember some of the things you say to her. When I give this advice, caretakers often tell me, "Oh, my God, Dr. Trujillo, she actually remembered me for a while."

Talking in this manner became such a habit for me that I even started addressing everyone like that. "Hi Mom, it's your daughter, Moraima, calling you from work."

"Would you stop that—I don't have atherosclerosis!"

Now, did you just rush by everything I suggested and say to yourself, "Oh, I already do that" or "Oh, I do that and it doesn't work"? If you do all this while your German is still semifunctional and you still have problems communicating, that's because people are unique. You can't always expect immediate results. People are not exercise equipment. You always have to take into account the human factor. Both patience and realistic expectations are required.

Unfortunately, you can't trust that your German will do what you say or follow instructions anymore. Keep reading and you'll see why. You also have to remember that even if you identify yourself, it might take some time for your loved one to process what you say. You might have to identify yourself repeatedly throughout the conversation. I learned that you can't force your dad to remember you no matter how much you want him to. Yes, I know he looks the same and sometimes even acts the same. He may only lose it for a few moments. Don't be fooled. Trust me, I know from experience. His brain is not working as yours is. You have to be patient and accept that he is sick. Don't get upset over it.

Let me give you a real-life example of this. Here's something that happened with my dad.

For most of his life, Dad took his medications on his own. But as we started keeping a closer eye on him, we realized he had started to forget his pills. "I took my medications already," he would say, even when he hadn't. You could argue with him until the end of time, and he would swear he had taken his meds. Mom would insist he hadn't taken his pills. In response, Dad became defensive and aggressive; he would pull out his journal and start scribbling in it. He believed Mom was undermining his position as man of the house by telling him what to do and how to do it—plus, he was convinced that he had already done it.

After a few of these bickering battles, I learned that if Dad said he didn't want to take the pills, it was best to leave him alone. Walk away. I would come back in a little while and say, "Hey, Dad, it is time to take these." I'd leave the medication in front of him with a glass of water. Then he would swallow the pills like a little lamb. It was as if his twenty-minute argument with my mom had never happened. He basically forgot that he forgot.

What did he need?

To take his medicine.

What did we want?

For him to take the pills.

Why didn't he want to do it?

He thought he had already taken them.

What was our mistake?

We argued, trying to convince him that we were right. We created a conflict.

The solution was to let him settle down. Allow time to pass so that your German can focus on something else and then approach them with the same request. Don't mention the argument, just (for example) place the pills in their field of view. At that point, taking the medication was just a reflex for my father. That's how easily suggestions in the environment can influence your German's behavior. A very high percentage of the time, Alzheimer's patients will forget what they were arguing about and cooperate. This way is much, much easier than trying to convince them that they're wrong.

There is an old joke that changes depending on when and where it is told. I was surprised to hear it here in the United States because I had heard it first in my native country of Cuba. To open the international borders, I'll give you the Cuban version here. A famous general (or dictator) and his lieutenant are driving their jeep past the yard of an insane asylum that is in the middle of nowhere. All the lunatics are outside playing baseball, running the bases backward. The jeep hits a large rock, which results in a flat tire. The lieutenant runs to change the tire. Seeing this, the inmates of the asylum abandon their game and start jumping on the chain-link fence, howling and hooting. This startles the lieutenant, who drops the lug nuts and loses them. The general is furious and screams, "Now how will we ever drive out of here?" The lunatics laugh at him and say, "You should take one lug nut from the three other tires to put on the spare." And as the lunatics start twirling in circles, they say, "*We may be crazy, but we're not stupid.*"

As much as I hate the use of the word "crazy," I hope you got the point. Yes, Alzheimer's is a mental illness, but Alzheimer's patients are not crazy; more importantly, they are not stupid. They will notice when something is wrong. They might not be 100 percent clear on what the issue is, but they will still notice. And they still have their pride.

In the case of my father, he was a very proud man. He always combed his hair, applied his favorite cologne, dressed neatly, and shaved every day—even if he was only going to bed. He held himself to his own high standard of what a man should be. One of his principles was that a man should always be strong and capable of protecting the women of his family. He never had any sons. It was just my sister and me. If he got sick, who would protect us?

After we initially took Dad to the doctor, I noticed that he spent a lot of time writing in his black work journal. He would never let anyone see it, not even little Nora, who couldn't read. But just like his wallet, he eventually started to forget where he left it. One day I found it and planned to return it to him, but of course, I was curious. *What was he writing about us?* It was the Pandora's Box reflex. You can't help yourself; you have to look.

Brush teeth and hair . . . make sure to put away the tools . . . at 5:00 come inside . . . put cigarettes in ashtray so wife doesn't nag you to death . . . the wallet is by the ashtray. He was keeping a list of everything he was forgetting. He had a daily schedule that covered everything he was supposed to do, down to the smallest detail—*remember to read this journal in the morning.* When I read this, I realized how much he was forgetting—and how much his pride wouldn't allow him to admit.

I'm willing to wager that before reading this section some of you fairly clever folks were probably thinking, *This doctor is not so bright. Why doesn't she just write things down so her father remembers them?* Unfortunately, Germans forget. They forget to check the list, they forget where the list is, and they forget that the list pertains to them! A list will work for *you*, but you don't have Alzheimer's.

My father knew he was sick. When he first noticed he was having trouble with his memory, I think he knew that there was something wrong. But his pride required him to hide his difficulties. To keep us from finding out, he began to withdraw from us. It was hard for him to deal with what was happening. All his life, my dad had been the man of the house. He thought his sickness was a type of weakness. His pride would not allow him to talk to us about his problem.

Family Dynamics

Remember that the person you are dealing with is still your parent. It's very easy for you to read instructions or find advice on what to do and what not to do. The tricky part is how to relay that information to your mom or dad. Yeah, you're just going to go right up to your mom and say, "I know I'm just the little kid you brought to life, whose diapers you changed, who you sent to school, but now you're going to do what I say because it's best for you." That should go over well.

And then you've got to have the guts to go to your mom, lay down the law, and tell her how it has to be. Remember how you used to be afraid of getting in trouble with your parents? The fear of that certain look they gave you? As it turns out, that feeling never goes away. There was a time my father said, "You're never too big for me to throw over my knee." And even though he didn't lay a finger on me, it was like I was seven years old again. Of course my parents aren't going to take orders from me. I wouldn't stand for that behavior from my kid. So how do you tell them there are things they can't do anymore? Unfortunately, there isn't a right way to give orders to your parents. They still know they are your parents, even if they are frail and senile.

This is why it's so important to remain respectful. You don't have to take charge of the person to be in charge of the situation. You don't have to tell them what they can and cannot do; you can assist.

Say your dad has started to show signs of dangerous behavior. First, try talking to the German about his feelings and ask for his input on the situation. There is a chance he will pull away and not want to talk to you about it. And even if he does admit there might be a problem, there's a good chance he'll forget what you're talking about halfway through the conversation. Try to include him in these conversations anyway.

Next, have the family sit down together—without treating the German like he is the problem. Remember, he is still part of the family. If you can, include the German; if not, try to have the meeting without his noticing. This may sound sneaky, but it's to avoid offending him. In this meeting, you should educate everyone as much as you can about dealing with Alzheimer's. Share what your doctor said; make a plan to ensure the German is always supervised; discuss the importance of avoiding conflict and the proper way to talk to a German. There is no substitute for a well-educated family when you are facing Alzheimer's.

The German's spouse faces a different set of challenges, especially if the couple has been together for a very long time. When a couple has been together for decades, as my parents were, they have learned each other's nature inside and out. They have an established routine—until Alzheimer's comes along. Then everything changes. Suddenly my mother no longer understood the person to whom she was married. The changes are painful. If the spouse doesn't learn how to adapt, a union that has lasted for decades can wear out.

A large percentage of partners of Alzheimer's patients begin to spend more time at home because of their spouse's illness. They'll cut back on seeing friends and family. Essentially, they display the same symptoms of withdrawal and isolation. Some of them are so embarrassed that they will never let anyone know they're married to a German.

My mother went into very deep denial after my father was diagnosed. She spent most of her time with Dad, so she saw him when he was high functioning. Then, suddenly, he would change; he would become confused and disoriented. In response, my mother took to the belief that "He's faking it! He only does this to annoy me. He's schizophrenic; he can't have another disease as well. He can't have Alzheimer's! We have been together forty years; he is not allowed to forget me!" At the same time, her pride kept her from exhibiting her sadness. She had dealt with my father's schizophrenia with fortitude, not tears. She didn't get sad then, and she wasn't going to now. Instead, her struggle manifested itself as anger.

My advice to spouses is to remember that your partner is sick. Alzheimer's doesn't care if you have a special bond. Alzheimer's disables the brain function of your loved one, but your emotional response to the disease doesn't have to disable *your* brain function. Use your knowledge and experience. Showing care and understanding in a stressful situation will bring you better results than crying or fighting. If you can keep in mind the fact that it is a disease that makes your German act this way, you will be better equipped to cope with those moments when his or her memory lapses.

Chapter 6

Sundowning and Other Symptoms

My mother might have been better able to cope if she understood the phenomenon of sundowning. Sundowning is a sharp and sudden change in personality that occurs when sunlight is limited. A person will seem completely normal, and then the sun starts to go down. The change begins with small but noticeable behaviors that might come across as tiredness. Confusion and disorientation set in. People who are sundowning don't recognize their surroundings or the people around them. They might walk around in circles or even wander off. They can't sleep. But when the dawn breaks, all these strange behaviors melt away in the warming rays of the sun. And the people who went through this change will never even realize it. They will get dressed and have breakfast, completely unaware of what transpired the night before.

Sundowning is brought about by the lessening of light and thus of stimuli. The brain becomes unable to focus on the activities of the day and gets lost in its own environment. People who experience sundowning often stop sleeping at night; some of them don't sleep even in the daytime. They don't seem to need much sleep at all, which can interfere with the rest habits of other people in the home.

Sundowning is a nightly occurrence. Once the symptom appears, it is there to stay. As Alzheimer's progresses, there comes a point at which the confusion also happens during the day. Unfortunately, it will always be worse at night.

Let me alert you to the hidden dangers of sundowning. As the sun goes down, many Alzheimer's patients lose their capacity to stay in touch with reality. They also forget what they need to do for their own well-being. Specifically, they often forget to take their medications or, because of sundowning confusion, flat-out refuse to take them. The reality is that they may have multiple medical problems (like heart conditions, blood pressure, etc.) that require medication or monitoring (such as finger sticks for diabetes). Other problems related to sundowning include wandering or bumping into things and falling because the person doesn't remember to turn on the lights. People experiencing sundowning also can become aggressive if they misidentify someone in the dark.

Lights, Locks, and Medication

You can help your loved one adapt to sundowning to some degree. Often sundowning can be managed with sleeping pills. When Dad developed sundowning symptoms, I couldn't do much other than try to clarify things for him. So I kept lights on throughout the house because he kept waking up at night. I made sure he took his medications so that he would sleep through the night because otherwise I had two problems: one, he was night-walking, and two, he would walk into other people's rooms and wake up them as well. I also made sure all the doors were locked at night to keep him from leaving the house. It was hard enough to find him when he wandered off during the day; imagine how bad it would have been if he did it at 3:00 a.m. and we didn't notice he was gone until the next morning. By taking those three little precautions, I avoided some major sundowning incidents. But the morning after that first major incident was still a rough one.

Signs and Symptoms

As we're already discussed, the "Big Three" symptoms of Alzheimer's are memory loss, wandering, and sundowner syndrome. We covered wandering first because chances are that you won't pay much attention to the memory loss until something big (like a wandering incident) happens. It's very easy to read a list of symptoms. It's a whole lot different when you experience these symptoms in real life. Like I tell my students, the list section of their textbook is just a guideline; you still need to read the whole book. You're still going to need to know how these symptoms look in the real world. Examples help, but the personal experience is priceless.

Here are some other symptoms to keep an eye out for in Alzheimer's patients.

Early Indicators

They start making mistakes when doing simple things they were once very good at—without noticing. They may dress unsuitably or put clothes on incorrectly. Maybe they urinate or defecate inappropriately. It's not that they're incontinent. They just really forgot that you have to get up and go to the bathroom.

Repetitiveness

They will keep asking the same question or saying the same thing over and over. If they have something in their hands, they may keep thumbing it or turning it. They'll start one action and then just repeat it, like a warped CD that skips back and keeps replaying the same five seconds. Other repetitive actions include pacing, losing things, talking constantly, and making repetitive noises like huffing, squeaking, or clicking.

Isolation

Like most things with this disease, symptoms of isolation are not 100 percent clear. In the beginning, my father's pride prompted him to withdraw from us. He isolated himself because he knew there was something wrong. Every time we brought up an issue, he felt criticized. Isolation could be a direct result of Alzheimer's, or it could be an emotional by-product of stress or fear of others' reactions. Because Alzheimer's patients don't want to deal with their memory loss, it makes sense that they try to conceal it and tend to avoid anyone who might say something about it.

Loss of Inhibition

As the disease progresses, the brain loses its concepts of social norms. Patients start doing and saying things that they previously wouldn't. Their attitude can become more brazen or flirty. They will confront people they wouldn't have challenged before. They may make inappropriate comments to someone they find attractive, and it won't matter to them if you are standing right next to them. It may be very embarrassing or funny depending on where you are.

Aggression

I don't think of irritability and aggression as symptoms directly connected with Alzheimer's. I see them as side effects, emotional responses to the frustration of living in a world you don't remember and feeling unable to control your situation. People generally become aggressive when they believe one thing but everyone around them adamantly says they are wrong.

Frustration on both sides can cause emotions to boil over, leading to arguments. But it's not the end of the world. It's better for you to simply agree with your loved one, no matter how far off he or she may be. Don't get angry.

One thing I've learned from experience is that anger in an Alzheimer's patient usually finds a physical outlet. When

Germans get angry, they spit. They spit out medication and food. They also bite, push, shove, squeeze, pinch, tackle, kick, scream, scratch, take things, break things, refuse to eat, and start using obscenities.

Aggression is considered a symptom because when Germans are angry, they do not handle conflict as the average adult would. The disease has worn away inhibitors and control functions. Therefore, they express their anger the way a child would. Of course, a large adult throwing a temper tantrum is a lot more frightening than someone who is barely two feet tall doing the same.

Let me restate my central point: You cannot argue rationally with this disease. Do not try to force a point to a brain that cannot process it. You will only make the situation worse. For example, if your dad has an aggressive outburst, do not antagonize him. Agree with him. Keep calm and try to guide him, gently, to where he needs to be. Please note that I said "where he needs to be," not "where you want him to go."

Yes, this is your family member, the one with whom you used to be able to reason—used to. But right now there is a disease in control of his brain. No amount of talking will convince this disease that it should believe what you are saying. Your best option is to prepare yourself now. Get educated, and within a relatively short time, you will be surprised to realize that AD doesn't surprise you anymore. You can handle this.

D ad wasn't the only one with pride issues.
I can't speak for my mother, but I can comment on her reactions to my father's illness as an outside observer. Mom was extremely old-fashioned. My mother always taught us that mental illness was something you didn't talk about, something to be ashamed of. But then, according to my mother, pretty much everything was something to be ashamed of. Yep, she was that old-fashioned. When I was young and my father had schizophrenic episodes, we would take him to the state hospital very quietly. That is actually a big credit to my mother, since many families just lock their "crazy cousin" in the back room.

My father suffered from mental illness for a long time. When I was little, my mother was the most stoic and courageous person in my eyes. She would manage the household without him whenever he had to be hospitalized. And this occurred in a time and place when married women weren't supposed to work.

We also lived in a very machismo society, and my mother was very attractive. There were men who came around when my father wasn't there. They offered her marriage; they offered her money; they offered her anything and everything. No matter what they offered, she would never let them in the door. She would walk by them on the street as if they weren't even there. For better or worse, she had married my father, "in sickness and in health," and they would be together till death parted them.

Then Alzheimer's added a new twist.

Dad was a funny guy even when he wasn't sick. He wore nice pajamas with long pants and long sleeves to bed every night. He would brush his teeth even though they weren't real. I have no idea how my mother endured.

On one particular evening, he woke up, probably needing to go to the bathroom. When he came back, he pulled the covers off Mom and said, "Lady, what are you doing here? Get out of my bed, I'm a married man!"

She looked at him in total astonishment. "Trujillo, what are you talking about? I'm your wife!"

"Excuse me, madam, I know my wife very well. You are another woman. I don't know how you got in here, but you better get out before my wife gets back."

Ever the devoted husband, he gently shooed this "strange woman" out the door without actually touching her so that his wife would not get upset. However, his wife was furious. The more angry and frustrated she got, the more she tried to convince him that she was his wife. Finally, he turned around and told her, "I do not sleep with prostitutes!"

From the other end of the house I could hear Mom's thunderous screaming. It was very, very early in the morning. My alarm hadn't even gone off. Half asleep, I stumbled toward this latest disaster. Nora watched from the floor, holding her stuffed panda over her head as if she were watching Saturday morning cartoons. My parents were oblivious to her presence or mine. They just kept at it. The more Mom screamed, the more frazzled Dad became. I cut in, trying to calm her down. Dad looked at me and screamed, "Get her out of here! Get her out of here before your mother gets back! I have no idea where she came from!"

He thought he was being an honest, faithful husband, but he didn't remember he was married to her. Maybe she had bed head. She probably looked just as bad as everyone else does when they first wake up. But he really didn't recognize her. I understand her frustration. Anyone would be upset when the person you have gotten into bed with every day for over forty years suddenly freaks out and says that you're just a hooker who sneaked into his room. However, instead of understanding that it was not really her husband talking, that there must be something really wrong with him, my mother thought, "I'm going to convince you that I am your wife. I've been putting up with you for forty years; you'd better remember who the hell I am."

I finally managed to calm her down. I took her to the kitchen to make coffee. She cried because she was angry and felt completely rejected. The first thing out of her mouth was, "The two of us makes one too many in this house. Either he leaves, or I leave!"

I had to be the peacemaker. "Calm down, calm down."

My daughter was jumping all around, asking, "Mommy, Mommy, why is everybody fighting?" I picked her up, took her back to her room, and put her to bed. She went out like a light. The biggest problem at that point was that it was still really, really early. It wasn't time to be up. Mom wanted to go get some rest, but she refused to get back in bed with a man who had called her a prostitute. My father refused to move from the doorway until the hooker left and his wife came back. Obviously, his wife wasn't coming back to the room.

I was at a loss. "Mom, just for tonight, go sleep in my room."

She pointed to her room. "That is my bedroom! That is my husband! And I have the right to go sleep there!" Oh, brother! It was a hell of a night.

Finally, Dad got tired and went back to bed. I followed him into his room, closed the door, and told him, "It's OK. She left."

"No, I did not!" I heard my mom protest. "I am right here!"

Oh, God help me, I thought. *What am I supposed to do?*

"He doesn't know who I am after all these years!" my mom went on. "I have cleaned his underwear! I have wiped his bogeys! I gave him two children! I've been with him in the good and the bad and the sick and the health for the better . . ." I must have listened to that wedding oath four times that night. She was voicing her frustrations and her inability to cope. She expressed herself all night.

Finally, my alarm clock went off. Mom had to let me go so I could get ready for work and get my kid ready for school. I was worried about leaving. I didn't know what would happen next. But what was I going to do? I couldn't call work and say, "Sorry, I can't come in today. My father forgot who my mother is, and I'm afraid that if I leave them alone together they'll end up killing each other.'

When Dad woke up that morning, he was in a little bit of a daze, but he behaved as if nothing had happened. My mom was frustrated. "Look at him, just pretending he doesn't know what he did."

But he really didn't know. My father's condition was deteriorating. My mother was ready to return to her old standby and ship him off to the institution. Understandably, she didn't want to be kicked out of her own bed every night, but at that time I was not willing to put him in a home. I was tired of having him in and out of institution after institution. I thought I could fix him. I thought I could control him. But my mother insisted that she was not going to let a man who had called her a hooker back into her room. Finally, I calmed her down by proposing a family meeting. I said we needed to decide what to do with Dad since he was only bad some of the time.

She looked at me. "Oh, that's because you don't know. I'm home with him all the time. You're not here. You're working. You don't have to put up with any of this!"

It isn't uncommon for relatives to come into conflict with each other over Alzheimer's. Say your sister feels overburdened because she is spending the majority of the time around the German, and it seems that everyone wants to dump the problems on her. Again, it is important to do everything you can to avoid conflict. If someone is unhappy because she feels she is shouldering the majority of the responsibility, you have to discuss it. You have to find a resolution everyone is comfortable with. I had a few options.

Plan A: Mom and Dad keep sharing their room and we all hope nothing like this happens again.

Plan B: Send Dad to a home.

But what do you do when no one can agree on Plan A or B? Create a Plan C. Try to find a creative alternative or compromise when no one can agree on the options available. We just had to put Mom and Dad in different rooms. But we didn't have any extra rooms in the house.

So I decided to build my father his own room in the garage, using the skills he had taught me. First, I had to clear out all the clutter. Then I had to take measurements and clean up all the grease and dirt. I laid a small layer of cement on the floor to make it even. Of course, my father couldn't watch any type of home repair taking place without jumping into the project himself. What, you might wonder, could possibly be worse than having your Alzheimer's-stricken father as your project boss? When he decides to bring in your six-year-old as your foreman. You might think that decision was Alzheimer's related. It wasn't. Giving project power to a person who can barely lift a paint can is a grandfather thing.

To be honest, having to move my father to his own room was such a painful experience that I've repressed most of it. But I do remember installing the air conditioning unit. I remember having to bathe my daughter afterward as she somehow managed to paint more of herself than the wall. But all in all, we had built a decent room. It had carpeting, a folding bed couch, and a personal TV for my dad. This was before everyone had a TV in every room in the house, so in a way, my father began the trend.

Chapter 7

Getting the Kids Involved

Alzheimer's affects the kids in a household because it affects the adults. Often, children want to be involved in everything. They might even try to think of a way to "rescue" their grandparent from the disease. As parents, we want to be strong in these situations to protect them. The truth is children can't do much to assist with the major things like medications or hospitalizations, but they still try to find their own ways to help. Seeing this can give parents courage. We gain strength from their spirit. So, how can you include the children as you deal with Alzheimer's in your family?

Sometimes you can't. Let's say there is a situation where you have to hospitalize your German and you bring the kids with you because you can't find a babysitter. Don't give them pointless jobs. "Oh, you want to help? Here, hold Mommy's purse while I fill out these insurance forms." Of course you will find yourself in situations where the kids will only get in the way. In those cases, just tell them straightforwardly, "You can't really help right now," or "You can help by staying still while I finish this," or "You can help by watching your brother while I take care of this."

Yes, they will pout and get upset; don't worry about that. In a hospital situation you have to deal with the big problems first. Afterward you can sit down and tell them, "I know you really wanted to help yesterday, and you did. Seeing how much you wanted to help made me strong enough to deal with all that doctor stuff. And believe me, that stuff is hard; there were lots of papers and big words. You behaved like a champ in that waiting room." Always praise children when they do something right. Let them know.

If young kids are going to be around sick grandparents, they can learn to help in other ways. Kids can read to their grandparents, sing to them, show them drawings, or just talk to them. If the grandparent is in a wheelchair, the children can (gently) push the wheelchair around the block (always with adult supervision, of course). You can make them the watchmen. Tell them something like this: "OK, this is very important. You're going to make sure Grandpa stays with you." (Really, you're just letting them play together.) "I have all of his medicines." (But don't point out where the medicines are.) "If Grandpa gets confused, looks tired, or starts acting funny, your job—and this is very *important*—is to run to me as fast as [insert the name of a favorite superhero here] and let me know." (Just a side note: be sure you pick a hero who moves fast.)

Remember, kids can be flighty, so emphasize the importance of their duty. You need to make certain that they will come to you for any reason. You'll see why later. And you're not really going to leave them alone. Kids may not always know what constitutes an emergency or be able to assess the severity of one. They might think they can handle it. Sometimes they'll come to you for no real reason, but it's better for them to overreact than to try to handle a real problem on their own. My family learned this lesson the hard way.

And there's one more catch: grandparents can give orders too. "Let's not tell Mommy that Grandpa forgot where the park was, and I'll give you a chocolate bar." Or they might suddenly get confused and take it out on the child. Keep watch from a vantage point or check in on them every few minutes. This way, both the kids and grandparents can think they're in control even when it's really all you. You're giving them power without giving them power. And it's not really about power; it's about inclusion.

Obligatory Disclaimer

Never let small children handle medication. I always locked the medicines out of Nora's reach and made it very clear to her that she was never to touch them. From my experience, no matter how obvious you think something is, if you don't tell kids, they won't know (and that applies to adults sometimes as well).

To give you an example, I know of one little girl (not Nora) who wanted to go faster on her bike, so she tried to hold on to a passing bus. Nothing happened; it was a slow-moving bus and she got busted before it went any faster. Her father was understandably upset, but she protested, "No one ever said I couldn't do that."

Kids are smart, and sometimes they get the idea that they can do a better job than we do. *Why do I need to tell Mom if she's just going to give him a pill? I can do that.* Don't let minors handle medicines! Keep medication safe and out of reach.

<hr />

Nora

Hello? Perhaps I should say something now. Hi, I'm Nora, and I thought I'd give you another view of Alzheimer's. After growing up around my grandpa, I see Alzheimer's a little differently.

Remember how in elementary school they would teach you about the human body with that song, "the leg bone is connected to the hip bone . . ."? Well, my mom taught me about the human body with a real human skeleton. When the "Just Say No" campaign started, I think she was one of the few moms who used a slide show. She had a habit of teaching me everything in excess of the main subject. She didn't hide from me the fact that Grandpa was sick.

After the night Grandpa tried to kick Grandma out of their room, Mom sat me down in the kitchen and said, "Nora, you may have noticed that Grandpa has been acting a little funny lately. That's because he is sick."

"OK, let's give him the pink milk."

"No, I don't mean sick like a cold. This sickness is in his brain. It makes him act silly sometimes, and it also makes him forget things and, sometimes, people. And he might end up forgetting you. Now, I don't want you to be scared; he's still Grandpa. He'll still play with you. But if you see him acting funny or confused I want you to come and find me or Grandma or Auntie. Do you understand?"

I nodded and that was it. Wait, that was it? No diagrams? No pictures? For someone like Mom, who had always been so thorough with my education, this little talk was way too simple. This must have been just one of her reminder sessions that she sometimes gave me when a certain subject was very important. It probably meant that Grandpa's illness was getting worse.

I already knew that Grandpa had a mental illness. But, since I had been born, he hadn't suffered any episodes. Sure, recently he had started to forget who Grandma was, but she was always cranky and never let you do anything. He still knew who I was. My young, naïve mind concluded that I must be what was keeping him healthy. That's when I got the idea that I was going to cure Grandpa. Together with my cousin, Michelle, I set about looking for a cure.

"Let's check the fridge," I suggested. There we found lettuce and carrots and other vegetables . . . all useless. If we wouldn't eat it, we sure couldn't give it to him.

"Look," said Michelle, pointing, "What about that? I-iro-on-be-er—Ironbeer! The man on the bottle has big, strong arms like Superman. This must make you stronger if you drink it!"

"Good idea, Michelle. I know, let's add it to Dr. Pepper. It's called Dr. because it has medicine inside."

"Yeah! What else do we need?"

"My teacher said that when she gets sick she eats chicken soup. Let's get some chicken. Oh, wait, I'm not allowed to touch the meats."

"Oh . . . I know! When my mom makes soup she uses these little yellow cubes. The box has a picture of a chicken on it. It's like a chicken in powder form."

I knew where that was. We gathered the chicken bouillon, the soda, and some cookies (because cookies always make everything better), but our scientific brains told us that we still needed something else.

Then Michelle came up with a brilliant idea. "I saw on TV where they made a medicine for the king from this tree and it cured him. Maybe we can find the tree in your backyard."

Genius! We gathered up our ingredients and my plastic kitchen play set and went to my grandfather. "Grandpa, can you take us outside, please?" Of course he wouldn't say no. Besides, we were about to cure him. As Grandpa set up his lawn chair, Michelle and I continued our quest. There really weren't any trees in the yard, but there was plenty of grass. We figured they were about the same. Into my little plastic pot we put the grass and the powdered chicken. We ate some of the cookies, but we made sure to put in at least two. Opening the soda cans with our teeth, we poured in the last ingredient and stirred.

"OK," I said, "it's ready. Try it."

Michelle looked at me in shock. "I'm not trying it. You try it."

I took one look at that mixture and knew I wasn't going to drink it. "No, I'm older and I say you have to drink it."

"No, I don't."

We both looked over at Grandpa. Michelle announced, "Grandpa, look what Nora and I made for you."

He picked up our little concoction with amazement. "Oh, this is very impressive, girls."

"We made it for you. Drink it."

Even though he was still smiling, his eyes seemed to widen. "This is all for me?"

"Yeah, it's to make you stronger, like Superman."

"Oh, good . . . what's in it?" he asked.

"We can't tell you. It's a secret."

"Oh." He tilted the edge to his lips and pretended to drink. "Umm, that was good."

"No, Grandpa, you have to drink the whole thing."

"But . . . I feel so much stronger already."

That's when we heard my mom. "Guys, dinner's ready."

Grandpa seemed very happy to see her. "China, come over here and look at what the girls made."

Moraima

From the expression on my father's face, I could tell he was up to something.

"Moraima, the girls are so smart they made a secret formula to make people stronger." He handed me a toy cooking pot so he could flex his muscles. "See how much bigger my arms are?"

"Yes, Dad, you definitely look stronger."

"I know, and I feel so energized. I think I may start flying very soon. You should try it." *What?* Oh, no. I had walked into a trap.

"Go ahead, drink it up. The girls made it special."

"Yeah, Mommy, try some," Nora said.

"Yeah, yeah, try some," her cousin added.

"Yes, Moraima. Don't disappoint the girls."

I looked down at the swirling brown fluid with pieces of I-don't-know-what floating around. "What's in it?" I asked.

With an evil little smile that just barely hid his laughter, my dad replied, "It's a secret."

As all these smiling faces stared at me, it occurred to me that I might just be poisoned by my family. I had to think of something quick. "Look over there! It's the circus!" Even Dad looked across the street. In that second I dumped the liquid behind Dad's lawn chair.

"Where's the circus?"

"Oh, they drove by so fast. But I saw them. And I saw the clowns and pictures of the elephants in the big truck. Oh well, I'm so thirsty . . . let me just have a sip of this." As I pretended to drink from the now-empty toy pot I thought to myself, *I can't believe they fell for the circus trick.* "Mmm. Wow, I feel better already. OK, let's go inside and eat." And as the girls ran past me, I overheard my niece say, "I know what we can use for our next experiment." Then I turned to my father. He was still staring at the street. "Pop, what are you looking at?"

As he turned back he said, "A circus just passed by."

Chapter 8

Medicines

There are no magic cookies that cure Alzheimer's. As of yet, there is nothing that cures Alzheimer's. There are treatments available that improve the condition. However, there's a twist. None of these medications really treat the disease itself. They treat the symptoms of Alzheimer's, giving the patient a better quality of life. Doctors believe that slowing the progression of the symptoms associated with Alzheimer's will slow down the disease. But there is no proof that these treatments stop the progression of the disease. The medications used for Alzheimer's are also prescribed for other maladies such as Parkinson's, Huntington's, and other forms of dementia.

As with all drugs, these can be misused and abused. They carry a risk of interacting poorly with other medications.

None of them should be used if you are pregnant or nursing.

Side effects include all the new symptoms or sensations that test subjects experienced after taking the medication. There is a low chance of experiencing intense side effects (including libido boost). If your loved one experiences any side effects, talk to the doctor.

This list is not intended for you to weigh your options and consider which treatment is best for your German; that's the doctor's job. I am simply providing you with this information so that you have an idea of what these medicines are and what they do. I don't want any of you explaining to the paramedics, "But I was only giving her the medicines I read in Dr. T's book."

Now that we have that disclaimer out of the way, I also want to remind you that you can't fix every problem with a pill. There is always the human element. Certain behaviors may be indicators of other problems.

Medications Used to Treat Symptoms of Alzheimer's

Galantamine
An acetylcholinesterase inhibitor. It blocks the enzyme cholinesterase from breaking down the neurotransmitter acetylcholine (ACh). Neurotransmitters are the chemical agents that relay messages between brain cells (also known as neurons). By stopping the cholinesterase enzyme from

consuming the ACh, this medication increases the amount of messages the brain can send, receive, and process.

- For mild to moderate symptoms.
- Brand names: Nivalin, Razadyne, Razadyne ER, Reminyl.
- Side effects: nausea, vomiting, diarrhea, weight loss, fatigue, dizziness, headache, depression, insomnia, abdominal pain, dyspepsia, and urinary tract infection.

Rivastigmine
Another acetylcholinesterase inhibitor.

- For mild to moderate symptoms.
- Brand name: Exelon.
- Side effects: nausea, vomiting, abdominal pain, dyspepsia, constipation, sleepwalking, loss of appetite, asthenia, headache, dizziness, fatigue, diarrhea, tremor, and depression.
- Available in patch form to lessen side effects.

Donepezil
This drug stops cholinesterase to promote the ACh.

- For mild to moderate symptoms.
- Brand name: Aricept.
- Side effects: nausea, diarrhea, insomnia, vomiting, muscle cramps, fatigue, loss of appetite, dizziness, depression, sleepwalking, weight loss, infection, hypertension, and back pain.

Tacrine

Another acetylcholinesterase inhibitor.

- For mild to moderate symptoms.
- Brand name: Cognex.
- Side effects: elevated LFT (liver function tests), nausea, vomiting, diarrhea, dyspepsia, myalgia, loss of appetite, and ataxia.

Memantine

The only medication currently on the market that is not an acetylcholinesterase inhibitor. A type of anesthetic, it works on the glutamatergic neurotransmitter system. This system is involved with the processing of information and the development of memories. The drug is supposed to help cognition, improve behavior, and enhance abilities needed to perform basic daily activities.

- For moderate to severe symptoms.
- Brand names: Abixa, Akatinol, Axura, Ebixa, Memox, Namenda.
- Generally well tolerated. Side effects: confusion, constipation, sleepwalking, dizziness, drowsiness, headache, insomnia, agitation, hallucinations, vomiting, anxiety, hypertonia, cystitis, and increased libido.

Why are there so many acetylcholinesterase inhibitors? They all do essentially the same thing, but in different ways with different chemical compounds. They also have different price ranges. Every person is different; your German might respond better to one medicine than another. Only your doctor can really say. Different people will also experience different side effects.

A variety of factors can cause poor drug interaction. Those forms you fill out at the doctor's office asking about personal information may be a bit embarrassing, but they are not meant to offend. They gather essential information to help doctors predict how a person's body will respond to a drug. You're hurting yourself if you lie about those details. I cannot stress enough the importance of an accurate medical history! This includes honest reporting about other medicines, sun exposure, excessive alcohol consumption, race, gender, past illnesses (including STDs that have been treated), certain foods, and environment. Even some pollens that you have contact with can have catalytic reactions to medication. Consider this: there are certain pills that are toxic for premenopausal women to even touch. This might not matter if you're a seventy-year-old Alzheimer's patient, but if you're the thirty-six-year-old daughter who is taking care of said patient, then you need to know this. And remember, Alzheimer's patients are taking more than just Alzheimer's medication.

Akathisia

With Alzheimer's meds you are likely to run into akathisia. Akathisia is a drug-induced, Parkinson's-like syndrome. Signs of akathisia include pacing, fidgeting, irritability, repetitive leg movements, hyperactivity, agitation, subjective distress, and dysphoria. Akathisia is more common than people realize and is often misdiagnosed.

Treatment for akathisia is very simple: reduce the dosage of the antipsychotic drugs causing the symptoms. But again, there's a catch. The patient might need some of these medications they're on desperately, especially in the cases of violent patients or those suffering from paranoia. So do you treat the side effects by decreasing the dose of the medication and risk bringing back the other symptoms, or do you keep them on the medication and risk neurological damage? Talk to your doctor about all side effects.

As a doctor myself, I can tell you that doctors don't react well when people come in thinking they already "know" what's wrong. Don't go busting into your physician's office saying, "He has akathisia. Fix him." First off, he may be a German, but he's not a car. Don't take a person to a doctor and command the doctor to "fix" your loved one. It doesn't work that way. There is no rapid solution or magic wand that doctors can wave to make everything OK. What will probably happen is that the doctor will change the medicines around and monitor how the German reacts. Essentially, the doctor is putting your German under observation. The doctor might decide to do this in the hospital or to leave the German with you and ask you to report what you see.

Be straightforward and specific when you talk to your doctor. Say something along these lines: "Doctor, I think my German has akathisia because of x, y, and z." The majority of misdiagnoses (in all fields of medicine) result from the doctor's lack of accurate medical history information. If Nora or my mother had gone to the doctor after my father experienced akathisia, they might have said something like,

"He's walking in place." A doctor can interpret a statement like that in many different ways. Akathisia may be mistaken for agitation, anxiety, drug withdrawal, restless leg syndrome, or any neurological disorder. It might even be associated with the existing ailment. The result of a misdiagnosis may lead to a change in medication that could have negative consequences, such as depression, cognitive impairment, aggression, and even suicide.

The more information you can give your doctor, the better.

Smurf

My father took Thorazine to help him sleep through the night. This drug is no longer widely used. Thorazine had some unique side effects. It changed Dad's skin tone to an almost metallic dark tan. This didn't really stick out to me until Nora started school. After a coloring project in which the children had to draw their families, Nora had some questions for us on the drive home.

"Mommy, why are we white and Grandpa is black?"

My mother, who was driving, almost crashed the car. She still managed to respond, "He's not black—he's sunburnt!"

"Mom, don't tell her that. Let me explain. You see, Nora . . ." I started to say.

"What is there to explain? I told her. He has sunburn. Right, Trujillo?" My mom spoke to Dad over me.

"I spend a lot of time outside in the sun," my father said.

"You see! End of discussion. He's sunburnt."

It is funny how even today people are uncomfortable discussing race—even when the true story doesn't have anything to do with race. I was not satisfied with giving my daughter a fluff story. That night I took Nora to my den, sat her on my knee, and explained. "The reason Grandpa looks different is because he takes a lot of medicines, and some of those medicines react to the sun, and that causes his skin to look darker."

"Why?"

"Because the medicines' reaction affects the pigment receptors of the skin. . . ."

"Why?"

"Because they're very strong medicines. The severity of his condition requires. . ."

"Why?"

Oh no, the endless stream of why. What had I gotten myself into? Trying to think of an escape, I turned to my books. "You know, it might be easier if I showed you." I found the right book and turned to the section about Thorazine and its side effects. Suddenly Nora gasped in shock. I had forgotten that the section had pictures, including one of an extreme case.

"He's blue!" Blue was Nora's favorite color. The questions continued. "Why is he blue?"

"Because he takes the same medicines as Grandpa."

"Why isn't Grandpa blue?"

"Because he takes a different amount."

"Will Grandpa turn blue?"

"No."

"Will I turn blue?"

"No, no, he turned blue because of the medication."

"What about my medicine, will it turn me blue?"

"No, Nora, yours are vitamins . . . they're chewables. They're not the same thing."

"They come in different colors. Will I turn those colors?"

"No."

"What if I only eat the red ones?"

"No."

"How about only the orange ones?"

"No."

"Can I mix them together to see if I turn blue?"

"No!"

"How do I turn blue?"

"You can't!"

"Then how come he's blue?"

I broke. I couldn't take it anymore. This questioning had gone on for half an hour. It was worse than dealing with a German who kept asking the same question over and over. "He's a Smurf!"

And just like that, it stopped. Nora was so captivated by the fact that she had seen a real Smurf outside of a cartoon that she was left dumbfounded. I took advantage of her stunned silence. "OK, it's time for bed. Go kiss Grandma and Grandpa good night." And she zipped out of the room. It was finally quiet. I was so proud of myself. Oh so cleverly, I had escaped the constant questioner. While I was enjoying the silence and putting away my books, my mother came in with a look of concern.

"What is a Smurf? Is it bad?"

"What? Mom, what are you talking about?"

"Nora just went to your father and told him he was shrinking into a Smurf."

Chapter 9

Supervision

When someone is diagnosed with Alzheimer's, they will need around-the-clock supervision. Yes, that will affect your wallet. Fortunately, there are better medications today than when my father first got sick. When treatment starts early, these medicines can help slow the progress of Alzheimer's symptoms and give the person a better quality of life. This in turn allows Alzheimer's patients to stay out of hospital care longer. Still, they will need supervision. Someone will have to watch them in order to make sure they are taking their medications, bathing, and eating and to observe any changes. The degree of assistance required will vary.

Some families will have a member who has the time to look after the German. This could be a spouse or another adult relative. Yes, it *must* be an adult. In the case of my family, my mother was the one who took care of our German in the beginning, but as the disease progressed, it got to a point where his care became too big a burden for her. She took it very personally when my father didn't remember her. Emotions boiled over and led to big fights. She was taking care of my young daughter at the same time. Then my mother got a brilliant idea. If she told my dad to watch Nora, he would keep busy and not bother her. If something went wrong, Nora would call her. She thought she was killing two birds with one stone. But that didn't solve all our problems.

Nora

I loved when my grandfather would sit me on his lap and tell me the stories of his life. He really only told me three, but those were the ones I kept asking to hear. There was the story about the haunted castle on the seashore. He was the only man brave enough to live there. Whenever he invited friends over, they would see ghosts and take off screaming. Grandpa's secret was that no one else realized the "ghosts" were just fireflies.

Then there was the time he awoke in the middle of the night to a strange sound. He went out to the beach and saw a mother turtle laying her eggs. So he flipped the turtle over, took the eggs, and ate salted turtle meat and eggs for a week.

But my favorite story was about the time he built a bridge outside his castle. The next day he used it to go fishing and wound up landing a six-foot hammerhead. Yes, a shark! He bashed its head in, salted the meat, left it out in the sun for seven days, and ate shark for a week. That story was my favorite because I used to believe that he caught the shark in the canal one street over from our house.

Then there was the story he told me on the day we went to the mall. I think it's a common bond between grandfathers and kids that they both hate being dragged to the mall. We detest it even more when we're taken to the mall to go shopping "for us"—when in reality it's Mom who's going to pick out all the clothes. And we're not even allowed to go to the toy store.

As my mother and grandmother debated which shirt would look best on Grandpa, he and I stood around, bored out of our skulls. We wanted to sit down, but there were no chairs in the store. Instead we managed to sneak away to the window display, where we sat behind the mannequins. We really wanted to go home.

"Tell me a story, Grandpa."

"OK. A long time ago I went fishing on a bridge that I had just finished building the day before . . ."

"No, Grandpa, I want a new story this time."

"A new one? Uh, OK. Let's see. Once there was a beehive . . . and inside there was a queen bee . . . wait, wait, where was I? There was a beehive with bees . . ." I noticed he was confused. He started shifting his legs around and kept going back to the beginning of the story. Eventually he just kept repeating the same sentence over and over: "There was a queen bee . . . there was a queen bee . . ."

When my mother found us, she didn't panic, but I could tell she knew something was wrong. "It's time to go home now" was all she said. Apart from being slightly happy about finally going home, my immediate thought was, *Uh oh, I broke his brain! I hope Mom doesn't know it was my fault.* I never did find out what happened in that beehive.

The next morning was Sunday, and Sunday was park day. I jumped out of bed to wake up the family so that we could get going. The first thing I saw when I opened the door was Grandpa, who was taking very small steps down the hall. It was almost like he had been walking in circles. But who cared? It was park day! I had already put yesterday's events out of my mind. The only thing that mattered now was getting to the playground. I grabbed his pajama sleeve with both arms and tugged like crazy. "Park, Grandpa, park, park!"

He just looked at me. "Who are you? Maybe you can help me. I can't find Nora; she's my granddaughter. She's about this tall, with black hair. I have to find her. Today is Sunday and I have to take her to the park."

As he spoke, I believed he was playing a game. In reality his mind was probably telling him that I was the neighbor's kid who had somehow snuck into his house. He was still himself but looking for me. To him, I was not Nora. It was a strange game. But I thought we were playing, so I went along with it. The only thing better than going to the park is playing at home before playing at the park. (Correction: birthday party

at park trumps all.) I took his hand and we went searching
. . . in really small steps. We went past my door, Mom's door,
the bathroom, and the towel closet. I crouched down like he
did and kept searching; I wasn't sure for what. By now I had
decided that he must have hidden a present and now we
were looking for it. We took such small steps that we weren't
really moving—it was almost as if Grandpa were walking in
place.

All that searching must have made some noise because
my mother came out of her room. Grandpa looked at her.
"Moraima, I can't find Nora anywhere."

Oh good, I thought. *Mommy is going to play with us!* Only
she didn't want to play. She told me to go to my room. I didn't
get to go to the park that day.

Moraima

The more incidents we had, the more we learned. We
realized that leaving Dad and Nora alone together meant
that neither of them would be properly supervised.

After several incidents, we also grew more careful about
Dad's smoking. He could only smoke in the backyard.
If he smoked inside, we would watch where he left his lit
cigarettes. Sometimes he would go into the kitchen to
make coffee, which he loved, but he would forget and leave
the coffee on the stove. We learned what to do if we saw
him heading toward the kitchen. "Oh no, we'll make the

coffee, Dad. Now get out of the kitchen. Kitchen is women's territory." Yes, I know I may have set the women's movement back with statements like that, but I didn't want my house to burn down.

We established a routine that worked, and we assumed we had everything covered. We still had an important lesson to learn: assume nothing. That soon became Dr. T's number one rule of thumb. Inevitably, a surprise would throw us off track.

In addition to working on Dad's daily routine, I had established a solid routine for myself. I came home at night, tired, was jumped on by hyperactive monkey child, took off my shoes, and put my jacket in the closet. My closet, being the closet of a woman, had more things to hang than the closet could actually hold. One particular night, I hung up my coat and *bang*! The pole broke in two. This made a big racket, and everyone came to see what had happened. What a mess. It was late on a Friday night, and my clothes were all over the floor. My mother helped me pick up my wardrobe and put everything on the bed. My daughter tried everything on. Soon all my clothes made a very big pile.

Without thinking about it, I said, "We need to find a carpenter to fix this tomorrow." Oh, boy, did I ever insult my father's pride.

"Excuse me? You want to hire a carpenter who will charge you fifty times what it's worth and do a very lousy job? When I am your father and I am the man of the house and I know how to fix this? No way! We are going to buy a replacement pole. I will show you how; it is very easy."

"Dad, Dad, it's OK. You don't have to do that. You're already retired; don't worry about it. A carpenter will come and fix it in a snap." Why did I even mention the carpenter again?

"Over my dead body!" It was a no-win situation.

Fortunately Nora came to the rescue. "Pizza night!"

Usually when you're arguing with someone and you're interrupted by a small child who is excited about something else, you feel like ripping your hair out. But this time Nora's interruption was the perfect save. Friday night was pizza night in our house. Nora didn't want to go to Home Depot because she wanted to go to Pizza Hut. "OK, Pop, we'll do all that tomorrow. Right now we have to take Nora to Pizza Hut. Tomorrow we'll get up bright and early, and I'll help fix the closet." That was a perfect sidetrack, but what happened the next day was entirely my fault.

Instead of going to Home Depot early in the morning when Dad's mind was a little bit sharper, I did everything else first. If we get up early on Saturday, my daughter thinks it's because we're going to have breakfast at McDonald's. So I took everyone to breakfast. And since McDonald's was right next to the supermarket, my mother wanted to pick up some things. And so on and so forth. It was afternoon before we finally got the replacement wood pole and went home.

Now the stick was the right length, but it was thicker than the old one and didn't fit into the pegs in the closet wall. "Oh, Dad, this is not the right size."

"It is the right size."

"No, Dad, it doesn't fit. Let's just go back and get a smaller one."

"What are you talking about? This can be easily fixed. All you have to do is shave a bit off the end and it will fit."

That sounded simple enough, so I got his chisel and hammer from the garage. "OK, Pop, tell me what to do."

He snatched the tools out of my hands. "I will never have my daughters do these things. Here, hold the stick." I took the end of the pole and held it in place. Before I realized what was happening, I saw the chisel coming from the wrong direction and being hammered into my left hand!

It was very, very stupid of me to hold the stick. I should have been more assertive and just called a carpenter. The truth was that I felt bad about hurting my dad's feelings. I also thought the task was simple enough that he could do it. But instead he drove a chisel between my thumb and my other fingers, all the way to the bone.

"Why are you screaming?" he asked. He didn't know! He didn't realize that he had physically hurt me or that I was bleeding all over the place. And to top all that off, he was ready to hammer again. I took away the hammer from him, and he got upset because I was "acting weird." I was in horrible, agonizing pain, and I had to act cool in order to avoid making him more upset.

"Dad, don't worry about it." As I said it, I was crying and not sure if it was because my dad really didn't know he had hurt me, or because of the pain from having the chisel stuck in my hand. His body was beside me, but his mind wasn't. The dad I had known most of my life would have said, "I'm so sorry, I'm so sorry" and tried to help me. But that man wasn't there.

So, still bleeding, I sat him down and told him to stay there. I took the chisel, the hammer, and even the stick, worried that if he saw it, he'd try to "fix it" with something else. I threw all those things in the bathtub and locked the bathroom door behind me so he couldn't get to them. Then I wrapped my hand in a towel and applied pressure. Dad started following me, asking if we could finish the closet, so I sent him to the backyard. I'm sorry if that sounds cruel, but I was bleeding profusely at the time—and he really wasn't helping!

My mother was cooking in the kitchen. She had assumed that the screaming she'd heard was me arguing with Dad. As long as she wasn't the one putting up with him, she preferred to ignore the situation as much as she could.

"Mom, I need some help."

"What happened now?"

"I need you to take me to the emergency room."

She finally looked up at me and saw the towel stained with blood. Just like that, she was flat on her back, passed out on the kitchen floor. At that point my daughter came in and saw her grandmother on the floor. I tried to hide the blood, but she was scared all the same. "Mommy, Mommy, Mommy, what's wrong? What's wrong?"

"Nothing, sweetie. Mommy just got a little cut. Just go back and play in your room."

"What's wrong with Grandma?"

"She's . . . sleeping. She's taking a nap. So let's let her sleep and you go play."

"But she's on the floor."

"She likes the floor. Don't wake her up. Leave her on the floor. Just go play in your room very quietly until I say you can come out." Then I realized that there was a trail of blood in front of her room. "Wait! Why don't you go watch cartoons instead?" Hold on, the living room with the TV in it was next to the backyard—where my father was tapping on the window waiting for someone to let him back in the house. "I know! You can play in Grandpa's room."

"But he's not there right now."

"Yes, but . . . you can wait for him . . . like a surprise . . . please!"

As Nora finally went to the garage, it dawned on me that the only other coherent person in the house was a six-year-old. I didn't want to drag Nora (who was already scared) with me while I drove myself, bleeding, to the hospital, but it was totally unsafe to leave her with my unconscious mother while my Alzheimer's-stricken father paced around the backyard, screaming that we needed to finish the closet.

So I called my sister. "Sis, I need you to come to the house because I need to run to the hospital." I didn't tell her that I was injured.

"OK, let me just finish washing the kids first. . . ."

"No, no, no, Sis! This is a very bad emergency. If I don't make it to the hospital, someone is going to die."

"Oh. OK."

I waited at the door until she finally arrived, all dressed up with all her kids. "So where's Mom?"

"Mom is flat on her back in the kitchen. Dad is in the backyard; I locked him out there. There is a chisel and a hammer and a stick in the bathtub. I locked the door so no one can get to them."

"Wait, what happened to Mom?"

"I showed her this." I opened the towel, now almost completely soaked in blood, and showed my sister my wound. She freaked out, which was no help to me. "Sis, calm down! I need you to look after Mom, Dad, and Nora!"

"But you can't drive yourself!"

"Look, this is my left hand. I drive with my right. And stop screaming; you'll scare the kids! If I don't get stitches soon, it's going to get a lot worse. Just take care of Nora, and I'll call you from the hospital!"

It was all just one big disaster. I finally convinced my sister I could drive and made it to the hospital. One of the nurses in the ER recognized me and moved me right back. They tried to find a plastic surgeon to take care of my wound so it would leave less of a scar. I said, "Listen, just stitch it up. I don't care if it looks good or not. Just stitch it up. I have to go home." I told the doctor the story and he laughed and laughed. At the time, I didn't think there was anything funny about it.

An hour and a half later, when someone finally came around to stitch me up, I suddenly heard a frantic, familiar voice. "Where is she? Where is she?"

Oh, no. My brilliant sister had brought all her kids, my kid, my father, and my now-conscious mother to the emergency room. She had reached the conclusion that I must be dead by now since she thought that all the blood in the house amounted to two or three pints.

"Sis, what are you doing? Get out of here. Take them home," I told her.

Then my father looked at me. "How did you do that to yourself?"

By now my face must have turned a new shade of red. I turned back to my sister. "Hello! Is anybody in there? Would you please take them home?"

But she and my mom just kept asking, "Are you OK? Are you OK?"

The doctor looked at me and said, "Now I see why you were in such a hurry to go home." He finished me up and I discharged myself from the hospital. I had to drive myself, my parents, and Nora back with my hand all bandaged up.

Dad still didn't understand. "How did that happen?"

I didn't have the heart to tell him . . . but my mother, however, had no problem letting him know. "You! You did that to her!" There I was, trying to keep quiet, and my mother started yelling at him and blaming him. "You hammered a chisel into your daughter's hand!"

"No, I didn't! I would never do such a thing!"

"You did! You did! You don't know what you're doing anymore! You are dangerous!"

"No, Mom, it was an accident." But she kept shouting. Then I had an idea. I started to moan, "Oh, it hurts, it hurts. Please, keep it down; the noise is causing it to hurt." And that worked. The rest of the ride home was dead silent. That was the quietest night because Dad went straight to bed without a sound. Even though Mom wanted to kill him, she knew I would play my "it hurts" card, so she stayed quiet. And Nora stayed next to me caressing my arm to make it better. Just as she dozed off to sleep I heard her say, "I'm sorry Grandpa cut you with the screwdriver."

After everything I went through so that Nora wouldn't know her grandfather had caused my injury, she found out anyway. I guess it had been easy for Nora to figure out since my mother had been yelling at my father ever since she regained consciousness. And Mom told him over and over what he had done. Of course he wasn't going to remember, but my daughter overheard everything.

So there I was, lying awake in bed. On one side of the bed my sleeping child held my injured hand. On my other side was a pile of clothes along with a mess of dried blood, which I would need to clean up the next day. All I could think was, *I really should have gotten a carpenter.*

My father was getting worse, but we were learning as we went. At least it was rare that Dad's mishaps landed one of us at the hospital; most of the time we were able to laugh them off.

I was getting ready for a staff meeting when my mother called. "I'm sorry, Moraima, but your father walked off again."

Oh, no. Everyone else was already at the meeting when I came in and announced, "I'm sorry, I can't stay. I just got a call from my mom. My father wandered off and I have to go find him."

My boss looked at me and said, "Again? Didn't he wander off last time we had a staff meeting?" I could feel my heart sinking. She was questioning me as if I were a kid who said the dog ate my homework.

"I know and I'm sorry, but I cannot stay."

As I turned to leave, one of my coworkers said, "Well, if he wandered off, I'm sure he'll pop up somewhere."

The way she said it was so uncalled for. I looked her dead in the eye. "That shows it's not your father." My look must have been intimidating because no one else made any other comments as I walked out.

That stupid remark soured my whole day. I drove home thinking about all the bad things the staff would probably say about me in the meeting and fearing I would have to face disciplinary actions when the cell rang.

"China, I don't know where I am. Come pick me up." It was Dad. He had actually checked his wallet and found the emergency contact card I gave him.

"Dad, where are you?"

"I just told you I don't know. Now hurry up, I'm hungry."

"Dad, calm down. Just tell me what street you're on. Do you see a street sign?"

"Yes."

"What street is it?"

"Stop."

"What?"

"The street name. Stop. The sign says stop."

I hit myself in the forehead. "No, Dad, a sign that has a number. It should be green and on the corner."

"Why do you need the number? I just told you the name."

I had heard jokes about new Cuban immigrants who got lost and gave "Stop" as the street address. I never had believed them—until now. So Dad wasn't clear about the concept of street directions. What do you do if you need directions but the person you're talking to can't give you any? "Pop, is there anything else around there?"

"No, nothing, just the redheaded girl."

"What little girl?"

"No, not a girl; the redhead girl with the pigtails. The place where they make the hamburgers. Can we eat there?"

He was talking about a Wendy's. There were only so many in our area. Now I had a clue about where he might be. "OK, Dad, besides the redhead girl. Is there a white building with a fence nearby or is there a store?"

"There's nothing but a parking lot here . . . on the other side there are stores. They have palm trees in the signs."

I knew where he was. I had to keep him talking to me. He was hungry and I was worried he would hang up on me to get food at the redheaded girl's place. I raced down to the Wendy's in front of Dadeland Mall and found him at the pay phone on the corner. As I got out of the car I wanted to scream at him. I wanted to tell him off because he had everyone looking for him and I was in trouble at work. It had been my idea to give him the emergency card, the card he'd said he would never need. And he was just standing there as if nothing was wrong. All he said when he saw me was, "'There you are. I've been waiting for you. It's so hot. I'm thirsty."

And just like that, I couldn't be angry anymore. He was hungry and dehydrated again. It wasn't his fault. He was the one who was sick. I took a deep breath. He looked at me with childlike innocence. "Can we eat something now?"

"Yeah. Here, let's go to Wendy's."

"Who's Wendy?"

That's when I really laughed. Before I had been scared and angry, but now that it was over the whole situation was hilarious. This kind of incident really focuses your attention on your German. These moments can be very funny if you don't take them too seriously. And when the German is gone, these will be the memories you'll keep.

———✦———

Another time I was working on a weekend and came home late. As I came in the front door, no one came running up to greet me. That was strange. It dawned on me that the house was a little too quiet. I saw my mother cooking in the kitchen and asked, "Where's Nora?"

Mom looked behind her, looked over to the living room, and then toward the door. "Oh, she must still be playing outside."

Sure enough, when I went out to the backyard I found Nora, completely covered in dirt and grass and bouncing on her toy horse. My dad sat nearby on his folding lawn chair, sunburned, dehydrated, and covered in little flowers. He must have been out there all day. He was so exhausted I had to help him get back in the house.

"Mom, bring me some Gatorade."

My mother walked in and noticed my dad's fatigued state. "What happened?"

"Mom, he's been outside all day. He's dehydrated."

"Well, he should have just come in and gotten some water."

"Mom, didn't you think to go check on them?"

"If there was a problem, Nora should have come to me."

"But I took care of him," Nora said when she realized my mother was throwing the blame on her. "I gave him flowers so he would feel better."

Kids do not make good supervisors. A hyperactive, sugar-fueled child doesn't realize that a much older person doesn't have the same stamina. Given the choice, my daughter would live in the backyard, but a full day in the sun was too much for my dad.

It was my mother who finally said she couldn't handle it anymore. We called a family meeting. My sister couldn't take care of Dad because she already had four kids, and there was another one on the way. I was constantly working; sometimes I was at the hospital for thirty-six hour shifts. But I didn't want to send my father away. I was raised to respect my elders and to honor my mother and father.

I came up with a creative solution: I would hire a helper to assist with the care my dad required. Unfortunately, my mother had a problem with everyone we looked at. "How's that one going to care for your father? She's almost as old as him. This one is too young. She won't know what she's doing. I don't like the look of that one. Are you joking? I'm not having someone that pretty around my husband. You can't hire that one; she doesn't speak English."

"Mom, you don't speak English."

"All the more reason to hire someone who does. I don't like this one; she doesn't speak Spanish. Moraima, that one has a boyfriend!"

"So?"

"I will not allow anyone who associates with men I don't know coming in here around Nora."

"Mom, I can't do a background check on their boyfriends or husbands."

"Then find someone who doesn't associate with any man. . . . Moraima, how dare you! That last person you interviewed was a lesbian!"

"Well, what did you want, Mom, a nun?"

"How dare you suggest that we pull a nun away from her congregation to work as a housekeeper?"

"Mom, we're not looking for a housekeeper, we're looking for someone to help care for Pop."

"And how can they care for your father if they can't clean the house? If I had a housekeeper, I could have more time to look after your father."

You probably know someone like this. We tried to do things her way, but no one was good enough. The ones I did hire all mysteriously quit on the first day, before I even got home. "Mom, what did you do?"

With wide-eyed innocence, she would say, "I don't know. I was just giving her some instructions, and she got all frustrated and left. We really shouldn't have someone so high-strung working around a sick man."

My thoughts exactly.

I went to the fridge to grab a soda to cool my agitation and found a screwdriver inside. "Who's been watching Dad?"

"Don't look at me! I was too busy watching over the new maid!"

Dad wasn't exactly innocent in this whole debacle either. I switched things around. Mom could cling to her militant specifications of cleanliness; the helper would look after Dad. But I was no longer surprised when I got home and found that the latest person I hired had quit. "Mom, what did you do this time?"

"I didn't do anything. It was your father that scared her off this time."

"Really? What did he say?"

"I don't know. I wasn't there. She just screamed something about a hammer as she ran out the door."

Oh. Apparently the confusion caused by having a new person in the house had triggered my dad's paranoia. And he didn't like having someone follow him around, watching him all day. It was not pretty. At that time, there were no professionals who specialized in babysitting Alzheimer's patients. This coupled with my parents' distrust of strangers put me in a tough spot. My idea was ahead of its time and too much for my family. They must have scared a dozen helpers out the door. People must have thought we were the Addams Family.

I was fed up with my mother's hysterics and thought to myself, *Fine, if she doesn't want any help, she can just keep doing it by herself.* About a week after that, Mom came up to me as I walked in the door after work.

"Moraima, we have a real problem." Amazingly, she had figured that out. "I caught your father trying to put Nora out of the house. He was about to push her out the door. He was talking all this nonsense about how she was the neighbor's kid. If I hadn't stopped him, he would have locked her out. Any pervert passing by could have kidnapped her."

"Mom, don't be so melodramatic. She would have rung the doorbell, and you would have let her in."

My mother gave me a stern look. "Tell that to your daughter, who is crying in her room. You go tell her that because I can't do this anymore."

Nora wasn't crying, but I didn't find that out because I went to my room to cry myself. I was out of options. "Honor thy father and mother." But by honoring my father, I was putting too much of a burden on my mother. Then I had to watch my daughter's heart break when the person she spent most of her time with started rejecting her. And thank God we had not yet had a major dangerous incident, but still, Dad was putting my family in danger. My father was incapable of attacking anyone. He would never hurt anybody. But I had a permanent scar from when he'd unknowingly driven a chisel through my hand.

What if one of my nephews asked Dad to fix something for them? What if the next cigarette he left sitting around did start a fire? What if next time he really did lock Nora out of the house? One of my strongest motives for writing this book is to share what I know now and what I wish I had known back then so that others won't have to struggle as I did. I wish the options that are available now had been available then. Dad might have been able to stay at home if I'd had more knowledgeable support.

As we learn more about how to deal with Alzheimer's, we've developed compensatory strategies to address memory problems. Such strategies include daily schedules to follow, written memos, a digital recorder, a centrally located bulletin board, a memory notebook, etc. Memory-retraining modules exist and are widely available for computer application though their clinical efficacy has not been established.

Additional techniques for managing memory problems include:

- Keep belongings such as keys, wallet, medications, and bills in one storage location.
- Use a notebook to record information and date the pages.
- Use a day planner.
- Post a checklist by the front door.

- Make a list of tasks for caretakers to check before leaving the house, such as turning off electrical appliances, picking up their keys and wallet, closing the windows, taking care of pets, and so on.
- Keep important or frequently used phone numbers on a list near the telephone.
- Write down all appointments immediately with times, places and contact phone numbers.
- Leave yourself voice messages as reminders and check them often.
- Use a timer when turning on the oven, stove, grill, or other electrical appliances that need to be turned off.
- Use a timer as a reminder of when to begin or end specific tasks; these tasks also may be written in a memory notebook.

Chapter 10

Assisted Living Facilities

My father was still a Trujillo, and any assisted living facility (ALF) would be honored and privileged to take him in. Or so my mother convinced herself. It was the housekeeper crisis all over again. No ALF was good enough. Finally I had to make the decision.

My advice to you is to check out the ALF you are considering as thoroughly as you can. Some would advise you to ask your doctor for suggestions; take that advice with a grain of salt. My personal suggestion is to ask someone with a loved one who has been in a facility for a while. If your acquaintance is happy with the services, take a tour yourself and check the place out at different times.

Remember that you have other options. If you've never visited a relative in a nursing home, chances are your idea of a nursing home is a vague concept based on popular culture and commercials. Most people have a negative perspective on nursing homes. The truth is, a nursing home isn't a place where you send old people away to live (or, as the bigger misconception goes, "where you send them to die"). A nursing home is a licensed medical facility that offers twenty-four-hour medical care. Usually patients stay in nursing homes only temporarily when they need rehabilitation. Patients often spend time in nursing homes after experiencing trauma such as a fall or a stroke. Their condition is not so critical that they need to stay at the hospital, but they are so frail that they need continued medical supervision and twenty-four-hour nursing surveillance. That's when they would be sent to a nursing home for a prescribed amount of time.

In case you are wondering, nursing home care starts at about $168 per day and averages around $70,000 per year. Don't count on insurance to help with long-term stays—nope, not even private insurance. Government assistance perhaps? Let me break it down. Medicaid and Medicare will cover nursing home costs if the patient is hospitalized for three days and enters a nursing home facility within thirty days of the original hospitalization. For the first twenty days, Medicaid/Medicare will cover everything. After that they'll switch to a daily deductible. If the patient hasn't improved after one hundred days, all coverage stops. Most insurance companies follow this template as well.

Only in the most extreme cases do patients live in nursing homes full time. These are patients who need constant medical care. This is not limited to patients with AD or to older patients—it includes anyone over the age of eighteen who is completely reliant on medical care. If a patient with Alzheimer's is still functional, a nursing home won't (or shouldn't) accept him or her.

So that's a nursing home. It's not the big building with rocking chairs on the front porch that you see on television; it's a clinic. Nursing homes are intended to care for your loved one in a manner that you and your family cannot provide. In a sense, though, you *will* be providing this care since you will be paying for it. Do Alzheimer's patients generally end up living in nursing homes? Only in the final stages when their minds lose control of all functions. (We'll discuss those stages later.) So if your German doesn't qualify for 'round-the-clock care in a nursing home but you can't provide the care and attention he or she requires at home, what do you do?

If you've ever passed a house with a sign that reads ALF, it's not because the residents are fans of that show from the eighties. An assisted living facility is a home that offers room and board to people who can't live alone anymore. They offer little or no medical care, but they cook meals; clean sheets; take care of utilities such as heat, air conditioning, TV, and radio; and in some cases offer assistance with bathing and dressing. They sometimes offer other amenities at an additional charge. The cost of an ALF ranges from $1,800 to $4,000 per month, not including extras. And no, insurance won't help with this one. Another option similar to an ALF is a resting home or retirement home. When people refer to "the home," they are usually thinking of these types of retirement communities. Cost is the same as rent for an apartment or condo.

If your German lives alone or if you want him or her to live with your family instead of in a home or ALF, consider the option of in-home care. There was a time that in-home care was only available to the rich. Now there are various, more economical forms of in-home care. These range from a full-time nurse to a nonmedically skilled individual who visits the patient for a few hours each day. If it is deemed medically necessary, in-home medical care may be partially covered by insurance or Medicare depending on your state's regulations. Nonmedical in-home care gets no coverage.

Keeping your loved one at home is the most affordable option and is least stressful for the patient. It is also the most stressful for the family. If you intend for your German to stay with the family, then you're going to need to make some changes. Learn from my experience; get the whole family educated and on the same page as early as you can. Work out a schedule so that someone will be in the home with the German at all times. Keep in mind that there will be days when Joe's car breaks down so he can't make it, or Mary can't wait for Ann to take over for her because she has to go pick up the kids from karate class. Prepare for those moments in advance when you're making a schedule. While you're making all these arrangements so that no one forgets, please be prepared for those moments when your loved one will forget you. As Alzheimer's advances there will be moments when patients not only forget their relatives' names but also become more disoriented, argumentative, frankly antagonistic, or just plain stubborn. In a confused state they may fall down or injure themselves in other ways. You have to learn to expect these moments. Remember, don't get upset.

Here comes that key phrase again: Avoid conflict. If you encounter opposition when you want the German to take meds, a bath, etc., don't insist. Chances are that if you insist, you will encounter more opposition and get frustrated, and we all know how that ends up. Just let the AD do its thing. Stop trying to get the task done; wait for your loved one to calm down, and they will forget the whole episode. After all, the important thing is to ensure that your loved one gets the care he or she needs even if you have to try again an hour later.

There is no law that requires you to put a family member with AD in the care of a nurse or doctor. So a caretaker can even be a housekeeper. For those of you who are thinking, *Wait, you mean I may have a medical excuse to hire a maid?*— yes, you do. Again, insurance won't cover it, but a housekeeper or maid can help in more than one way. For one thing, they can take over the maintenance of household duties so that you can focus on taking care of your German. Or you can hire someone as a companion, kind of like a babysitter, to watch over the German when the family is out. The job would include supervising medicines, preparing meals, cleaning up, and possibly driving the German to appointments. In more advanced cases of AD, a companion's duties would include changing diapers and cleaning up afterward as well as helping patients out of bed and gently encouraging them to move around so that they don't develop bed sores.

Another option to consider is a medical nurse. These nurses come to the house on a regular schedule and can handle a variety of tasks depending on your loved one's conditions. Their duties can range from checking blood pressure or blood sugar levels every few hours to monitoring medications and making sure the patient is eating, sleeping, and bathing.

I'm a big supporter of the senior center or what many of my patients call the "Little School." Senior centers, which are like day camp for seniors, have become popular in recent years. Centers work with nursing homes, ALFs, and private families. These day programs sometimes offer bus services. At the local senior center, your loved one will enjoy a variety of activities like games, crafts, parties, and occasional supervised field trips. These creative activities not only encourage stimulation of the brain but also provide opportunities for your German to meet new people. The "Little School" or senior center trend has caught on substantially. Many churches, schools, and YMCA locations offer senior day care; some programs operate independently as private senior centers. It is a shame, but this is also not covered by Medicare or insurance.

My father didn't want to go to a nursing home. There was nothing we could say to convince him otherwise. He protested, "You promised you would never put me in a home!" He was right—I *had* promised, and every word he said ripped at my heart. But I had run into a wall. My family could not offer the care he needed. Instead of dealing with the problem, my family let their emotions get the better of them, and Dad ended up paying the price. The only way I could make it up to him was by finding the nicest place possible. He didn't really appreciate that sentiment at the time.

Mom was the one who packed all of his things. She just grabbed everything by the armful and threw Dad's belongings into his suitcases so that she wouldn't see. She wanted to rush through it. We told Dad that we weren't abandoning him; we promised to visit every week. That didn't make a difference. We had broken our promise about putting him in a home, and visiting once a week was not the same as seeing him every day. To Dad, it felt the same as if we were abandoning him.

I kept remembering all the times I had passed harsh judgment on people who put their parents in nursing homes. Now I was one of them. It's easy to feel morally superior when you haven't been forced to watch someone you love slowly deteriorate until you are forced to make a decision. When we feel guilty, we either reprimand or excuse ourselves. You might criticize yourself or turn your anger outward and blame others. You may find yourself thinking of shallow individuals who sent their family members away for the wrong reasons. *At least I'm not like those creeps. I put mine in a home for the right reasons.* I want you to know you don't have to feel bad if you have to place your German in an ALF. The truth is that there is no "right" reason, only necessary reasons. These necessities may be medical or financial. Your reason might be "I don't want him accidentally hurting any of the children with a hammer." But I don't want your reason to be "he can't stay in this house because it's tearing the family apart." That was one of my reasons because there was no one to educate my family.

Nora

The day that we took my grandfather to the home is not a day I like to remember. I do remember that after the experience, I grew disillusioned with cartoons. Every Saturday it was always the same thing: "True love conquers all." They all said it. Strawberry Shortcake, He-Man, even the talking pillow people. Cartoons say that the people you love will always love you, and that no matter what terrible thing happens, love can always fix it. Well, I knew better. It didn't go down that way.

At first I was completely against the idea of putting Grandpa in a home. It was wrong. It was like throwing him away forever because he was acting silly. But then he didn't know me anymore and it was different. I was the grandchild who lived with him. I was the one he was always looking for, but now he didn't recognize me. I'm ashamed to admit it, but sometimes I hated him in those moments. But even then, I didn't want him to go to a home.

I remember the drive that day. It seemed very long, the home very far from our house. We pulled into the curved driveway of a residential house. It was yellow with a small chain-link fence on one side—the side where Grandpa was going to live. He actually had his own private door to the backyard. Mom went through the motions, showing us what a nice place it was. It had a big yard with a big wooden deck overlooking the canal. There were birds in a big cage outside and a barbecue. Then we went to his room—a little room with a little bed and a little TV set. It seemed so hollow. This wasn't where he belonged. He didn't want to be there; even I could see how upset he was. I had to do something. I had to save him.

Back to the cartoons. Every time the evil sorcerer puts a spell on the hero, the princess saves the day by reminding the hero of their great love. Just in the nick of time the evil spell is broken and the hero wakes up. I thought I just had to make one last-ditch effort to break the spell and Grandpa would come to his senses and hug me like he always did, and we could go home, to our real home. I ran up and hugged his legs as tight as I could and yelled, "Grandpa!"

I couldn't even finish that one word before he started screaming at me. "Who the hell are you? Why are you still following me?" My mother grabbed me by the back of my shirt and quickly pulled me away. As my grandfather kept screaming, I stormed out of the room. I marched angrily to the car and sat with my arms crossed until my mother came out to talk to me. I don't remember what my mother said, but I was so angry that, more than likely, I didn't give her a chance to talk. "I don't care!" I remember saying. "I hate him! I want to go home! And I never want to see him again!" My mother didn't answer me because now Grandpa had started screaming at Grandma, and my mother had to run back inside to break up the fight.

Remember how all those cartoons end? The spell gets broken, the evil sorcerer is killed, and the good guys live happily ever after. Turns out that's not how it goes. But I didn't realize that at the time. I thought cartoon characters deserved their success because they were always good. So the only explanation was that I wasn't good enough. Grandpa didn't love me enough to remember me.

Chapter 11

Kids

As a mother and a psychiatrist, I've come to realize that it is not always as difficult for kids to understand as it is for parents to explain. Sometimes we just don't want to tell them. Other times we think they won't understand. When you're the mom, it's easy to forget how the mind of a seven-year-old works.

I didn't have much of a childhood. By age eight I had to help maintain the house. When I had Nora, I told myself I was going to give her a better life than I had known. I was going to make sure that she had all the education and opportunities that hadn't been available to me. But at the same time, I taught her to believe in fairies and unicorns and told her that kisses could cure boo-boos. I believed children would naturally outgrow

Santa Claus by age ten, so I kept telling her Santa was real. Imagine my surprise when she still believed at twelve.

As her grandfather's disease grew worse, I wanted her to be prepared. I taught her everything I knew about the disease, which really wasn't that much at the time. She was a smart kid; she understood he was sick and knew it made him act silly sometimes. The problem with kids (and teenagers) is that when they know a little, they think they know it all.

I didn't realize that Nora measured her grandfather's love by his recognition abilities. Throughout his illness, I was the one person that my father could always identify. It hurt Nora that he could recognize me and not her. She was very understanding of his ailment until it affected her personally.

Young children and teenagers react in many different ways to watching their grandparents develop Alzheimer's. Some take it better and some take it worse; it really depends on the individual and the situation. If the disease emerges when children are very young, they may grow up completely oblivious to the situation. To them, grandparents have always had Alzheimer's, so it's nothing new. Older children who must watch as their grandparents begin to deteriorate will take it harder, especially if they have shared a close bond with their grandma or grandpa. It comes as a big shock when the person who once showered you with attention no longer recognizes you or when all the attention you used to receive from your family now goes to your grandparent.

Alzheimer's takes the most recent memories first. Memories of grandchildren are often the first to fade simply because the children have been around for a relatively short time. If your loved one shares a very close bond with the grandchildren, these memories may in fact be very deeply embedded, but children grow and change. The grandparent may hold on to just one memory out of all the rest as if holding on to a photograph. For example, a grandfather may picture his granddaughter as a laughing child with curly hair on a swing. Kids grow fast. Ten years later, the same grandchild will come to visit and say, "I'm going to college." Grandpa will compare the photo in his mind with the grandchild standing in front of him; in his mind, the two don't match. Even when only a little time has passed, a very small difference can be enough to cause that dissociation. The child might look the same, but when Grandpa refers to the photo in his mind, he sees his granddaughter on a swing in the park. If the child is sitting in front of a television set, his faulty memory tells him, "Yes, you have a grandchild, but this can't be her. She's at the park on a swing."

Nora

Mother always said I was a smart kid. But there's a lot that even smart kids don't understand. Perhaps you think, *My kid is very intelligent and advanced for her age; she'll understand.* But unless your child has been featured on the Discovery Channel or is a licensed psychiatrist, you might hit a snag. Even if your child understands the facts or even if she's a supergenius, relating to a grandparent with Alzheimer's presents big emotional challenges.

Think back to when you were a child. The world was very small. It was made up of only what you had experienced yourself. You had heard of places like China, Africa, and Mexico, but unless you had seen them, they were impossibly far away. Children see the world only as it relates to them.

A child measures illness by her own personal experience. Kids learn that if you fall down, you can go to Mommy and she will kiss it and make it better. I used to reason that if someone got sick, you sent them flowers and that was how they would "get well soon." Have a cold? Drink this, get better. Something worse? Go to the doctor, get a shot, and get better. The concept of a sickness that never goes away, something that even Mom can't fix, is very hard for a young mind to grasp.

That's just the way kids think. It's not that they're dumb or simple; it's the opposite. They're logical enough to calculate using their experience, but their experience is limited. And trust me, very few cartoons explain the truth about Alzheimer's or tell you that sometimes life is sad. To be honest, you wouldn't want your kids watching educational cartoons that make them cry. No, you want them watching happy animal shows where the fuzzy little bunnies don't get torn apart by hungry foxes.

Children are smart enough to ask questions that adults don't have answers for. And they're so creative that if they don't get an answer, they'll come up with one. Children process things with images. Tell a child that Granny has a disease in her brain and that child might visualize a little monster living inside his Granny's head. Of course his response will be, "Why can't you just get it out? Why can't they get better?" If you explain to a child that Granny is sick, that there isn't any way they can help and to just leave it to the doctors and grown-ups, they're not going to buy that. Kids have a mentality that grown-ups never listen to them.

You may not always know what to say, how to say it, or if they're even listening to you, but say something. Explain why Grandma or Grandpa had to be placed in a facility; remind your children that the decision has nothing to do with them. That none of the bad things that are happening to their grandparent are their fault. That it is a sickness that makes their grandparent act differently. That if they have any questions, it's OK to ask. Remind them that even if their Grandpa doesn't recognize them, that doesn't mean that Grandpa doesn't love them.

Another piece of advice: avoid esoteric rationale. Kids will write to Santa Claus, wish upon a star, or cast a magic spell, believing it will cure their grandparent. It's a very hard blow to them when these methods don't work. If you notice them trying to contact the fairy princess, nip it in the bud quick. Explain that Granny's sickness is of the medical, not magical, realm. Santa Claus doesn't fix these problems (he doesn't take insurance). Otherwise kids will be disillusioned when they expect their favorite wizard to show up and solve everything and it doesn't happen. So just steer them away from the magical quick-cure concept.

Accepting the truth will hurt, but they will understand it someday. Don't worry—this won't be a permanent emotional scar that will leave them traumatized forever and require years of therapy. It might be more upsetting for parents to watch their children process difficult emotions. That's right—this whole section has really been for the adults more than the kids. Children will be sad for a while, and then they'll go on to something else. Eventually they'll understand . . . when they get older. And even if they hate that answer, it's the truth. They'll just have to wait and grow up a little before they fully understand. By then, they might learn not to take it so personally.

When you're a kid, one thing is true: If something bad happens, it's always your fault. Whether it's a divorce or a disease, somehow you managed to cause it. At least, you tend to think that way. I started to review things in my mind. Grandpa got worse after I asked him for a new story. The mental powers required to create a new story must have been so strong that they broke his brain, I reasoned. All my cures were stupid too. How could I believe that you could cure someone with cookies? The children on television always managed to save their grandparents, but it didn't work that way for me; therefore, I concluded that I had failed in my duty of keeping Grandpa healthy. And now he was in a home. In an attempt to comfort me, my grandmother explained, "We had to send him away because he is not well and he gets confused sometimes, and we don't want him to do anything that might hurt you."

So it was my fault that he was in a home. They sent him away to protect me because I couldn't protect myself. But at the same time, Grandpa didn't care enough to recognize me.

I shouldn't care for him either. But for all that, as angry as I was at him, why was I still sad that he was gone?

It was strange not having my grandfather in the house anymore. Yes, I was mad at him, but I forgot about that when I would wake up in the morning and look for him. Most people don't remember their first cognitive memory, the first thing they were consciously aware of doing in their whole life. My first memory was of getting out of my bed, running to the living room where my grandparents sat in their fuzzy red chairs from the seventies, and knowing that this was Grandma and this was Grandpa. Perhaps that routine was just so ingrained that it was hard to break. For a long time, I would get up and run into the garage only to be reminded by Grandpa's empty chair that he was gone.

Somehow Grandma got the notion that I kept going to the garage because I liked hanging out there. She then came up with the brilliant idea of converting it to a playroom for the grandkids. Soon all my toys (along with the exercise bike my grandmother never used) were moved into Grandpa's old room. At first I was against the idea. There was a type of creepiness attached to it. To a certain degree, I think I started to believe that my grandmother was putting me in the garage because I was the next to go.

The room might have been cheerier if they had painted it in brighter colors or put up Disney posters. But at the same time, that would have felt wrong too. I think my mother had the same feeling that I did: repainting and redecorating would have been like trying to erase Grandpa. Instead she kept his things in there. It wasn't much: the sofa bed, the old wooden end table with the TV, and the metal tool shelves that were now filled with my dolls and stuffed animals. She said something along the lines that a part of him was still in the room and she was giving me his room and his furniture so that I could still be close to him. Closeness. How do you have closeness with someone you can't get close to?

I didn't understand what my mom meant about Grandpa being in the room, but it was actually a good thing that she said it. The idea of feeling close to Grandpa wasn't something I pondered with philosophical intensity. For crying out loud, I was seven! And now I had my own television. I could watch cartoons while sitting upside down on the couch with my shoes on. I could get away with it. This was a room that was blocked from adult supervision. Then I realized that the couch I was sitting on used to be Grandpa's bed. There was that creepy feeling again. But while hanging upside down, I caught a glimmer of something shiny on one of the lower shelves. It was an egg-shaped glass paperweight that got left behind when my grandfather moved.

"It's a Grandpa piece," I thought. No, a Grandpa piece was not a piece of furniture; I really thought this was a piece of my grandfather. See, when my mother said that a part of Grandpa was still connected to the room, I really believed that she meant a piece of Grandpa. Like a spirit version of my grandfather was inside the walls and was watching, hence the creepiness. This glass egg was a physical portion of my grandfather's essence lingering in the walls.

Continuing my exploration, I found a soapstone crocodile and a button. Even though they weren't toys, I hid the crocodile and the egg among my stuffed animals. The egg had a propensity for falling and cracking, but for all its cracks, I never threw it away.

It wasn't until Christmas that it really hit me. It was only one person less, but the house suddenly felt so empty when I started opening Christmas presents. Mom was tired from working the night before, and my grandmother was the type of person who believes you shouldn't play with your toys because you might break them. Christmas morning made me feel all the more the absence of Grandpa, who would always play with me.

One benefit of growing up in my family was that you got two Christmases. In the Cuban culture December 24 is the sacred night of Christ's birth. That night you have the big family dinner and rejoice. It's not until January 6 that the kids get presents. *El Día de los Reyes Magos*, or the Day of the Three Wise Men, celebrates the day the Three Kings finally reached Bethlehem and presented baby Jesus with his gifts. Every year on the night before Reyes Magos day, my cousins and I would collect grass and put it in buckets "for the Wise Men's camels." Hey, if we gave cookies to Santa and grass to his reindeer, we were going to do the same for the Magi and their camels.

But the first year we celebrated without my grandfather was also the first year that I had to go to school on January 6. Every year since I had started school, our special day of celebration had always fallen on Friday or on the weekend.

It was Reyes Magos day and they expected me to go to school! There was only one present under the tree. It was the orange, duck-billed dinosaur that I wanted. I kept him under my arm while my mother and grandmother rushed to feed me, dress me, and get me out the door. As they shoved oatmeal into my mouth, I thought about how Grandpa was not there—but he never really bought me any presents. He gave me presents, but I knew my mom was the one who had bought them. I was also starting to suspect that it was highly unlikely for camels (even magic camels) to shrink small enough to fit through the security bars on our windows. After pondering the matter, I concluded that *Grandpa is not here, but if he were, Orangey* (my new dinosaur) *is the present he would have given me.*

I still have the broken egg and Orangey the dinosaur. In fact, I keep both inside the wooden house that Grandpa built for me. The little house also holds jewelry and perfume that I have bought for myself on his behalf. After all, he would want me to have a Merry Christmas.

Moraima

When you are the mom, you don't think of things the way your child does. Sure, I could tell when Nora was sad or happy or when something made her angry, but I never knew she believed that Grandpa was in the wall. Children have a logic that is very unique, and it's much easier for them to have a concept for company than for an Alzheimer's patient.

Don't laugh; adults do the same thing. It's just easier to point out in children. Adults talk about their Germans with affection and think about them all the time. But then they don't make time to visit. Does this sound a little too familiar? Why don't they visit? Because it's uncomfortable. It's disappointing to spend all week recalling that time you went deep-sea fishing with your dad, the excitement when he caught a marlin with such bravado. Then you go for a visit, and instead of this manly angler you see a lethargic man who doesn't recognize you sitting in a chair twirling tissue paper in his hands. It can be very frustrating if you try to remind him of that fishing trip and either he doesn't remember or his AD is so advanced that he rambles on like you're not there.

Teenagers

Teenagers, on the other hand, have a better understanding of illness than young children, so it's easier to discuss these difficult topics with them—at least with regard to the facts. Unlike small children, they won't blame themselves because they understand the basic concept of disease. And they won't try to fix it either, because they've outgrown the hero phase. They generally don't take it personally, but sometimes they still get upset.

Many teenagers are wrapped up in their own personal concerns. Those are the "whatever" kids. Maybe they didn't like Grandma. Perhaps Nana was a nag. Having to go to her house every Sunday was a chore, something you had to do even if you would rather go out with your friends. As parents we tend to get angry because we feel our teens are abandoning their families in a really shallow manner. We say we are going to handle this as a family, but our teenagers would rather be playing *Guitar Hero*. This is not to say that our children don't care; it's often easier for teens to brush off their sadness and anger than to feel these confusing emotions.

Remember that children feed off the emotions of the adults. If visiting a sick German upsets you, your emotion will rub off on your kids. Just as young children can give us strength with their spirit and willingness to help, they can also get depressed when they accompany a parent to visit an Alzheimer's patient and they notice that the parent doesn't want to be there. So if you don't want to go, they don't want to go. This reluctance becomes more apparent in teenagers because they can vocalize their opinions very well. Also, by the time your children reach their teens, there is a very good chance that they've experienced an unpleasant incident as a result of Alzheimer's (Grandpa forgot me again). Their reluctance to visit the German might upset you. After all, even though you don't want to go, you brought your kids along to give you strength and support. But they pick up your reluctance and don't want to go either, and now you're stuck with a cranky teenager. It is easier to criticize their attitude than to admit your own feelings. Visit days can turn into a vicious cycle of frustration and avoidance.

I was very lucky with my daughter during the "terrible teens." She never gave me much trouble, but she did go through that phase where she didn't want to visit her grandfather. Though she had outgrown the "I'll hate you forever for getting sick" phase, I knew she still had some residual heartache. The mind of a young child reacts with emotions, and the easiest emotion is anger. But as knowledge sets in, the anger starts to fade, leaving sadness in its place.

At first I made Nora come with me on my weekly visits to my father. It upset her when her grandpa didn't recognize her. "Don't be sad," I would console her. "We'll go back inside in two minutes and he'll know you then." But as she grew older and more despondent I gave her a choice: "If you want to come with me on Saturday, we'll all have a great time, or you can just stay here." She chose to sleep in. I would ask and beg. "Please, Nora, it means so much to me. I would really appreciate it. I'll take you to the mall afterward."

It worked a few times, but one day she just turned to me and said, "What am I going to do there? I just stand there and do nothing. He doesn't recognize me. The times he does talk to me he's telling me about me without knowing it is me. And all I can do is smile and nod. And what's the point of me going if he's going to forget that I visited him the minute I leave?"

I didn't get upset. Well, maybe I was a little upset, but I kept it inside. And she had a point. Though teens may understand what is happening to Grandma or Grandpa, that doesn't mean they won't be saddened or depressed by seeing their grandparent's condition. What might come across to us as rebellious indifference is just their way of masking their concern.

Nora

Mom is overcomplicating the emotional logistics of a teenager. Short version: I didn't go because he didn't recognize me and it was boring.

Moraima

Or they could just be bored. It's a little hard to know that when teenagers don't talk to you. Again, it might be a little hard to understand how a teenager feels if they don't want to communicate their emotions.

Nora

Yeah, because teenagers love nothing more than sitting down with their parents and talking.

Moraima

Fine! I get it! It's not cool! If I make you go, I'm being a drag. If I don't make you go, I'm depriving your grandfather of additional family support. If I try to talk to you about your emotions, I'm a nag or whatever the latest slang is. But how am I supposed to know your feelings about the situation if you don't tell me?

Nora

I did tell you. I told you I didn't want to go because it was boring.

Moraima

Teenagers! But she did tell me. And even though she denies it, the answer she gave me said a lot more. The day she turned around on me and spewed out all her reasons for not wanting to go, she was clearly upset. So she didn't want to go not only because it was boring but also because her grandfather's memory loss made it difficult to have a real connection and that upset her. Of course it's boring when you can't interact, although I'm sure Nora is going to pop in any moment and say she was upset because I kept asking her to come with me.

So how do you get a teenager to visit her sick grandparent without getting bored? To motivate my daughter to visit her grandfather, I used her favorite classes in school. She had just started drafting and shop, and her favorite subject was history. So I got her interested in our family history. My father had lost most of his short-term memory, but he still had the majority of his long-term memory. In Cuba, he had worked as a draftsman. There were stories from before I was born that only Dad knew. Fortunately, Nora had learned about the preservation of history in school (if we don't learn from the past . . .) so she realized that if anything happened to her grandfather, all that history would be lost forever.

That's when I hit a snag. Nora had grown up enamored with her grandfather's stories, but now she was old enough to doubt them. My dad used to tell her about living in a castle, but now she had started to study history. "Mom, there aren't any castles in Cuba."

So I added a chapter of my father's stories that Nora didn't know. "No, there aren't any castles, but it was to your grandfather. When he was a young man, he set out to earn a living, but he had nothing. He was essentially homeless. That's when he found 'the castle.' In reality it was an abandoned military post from the Spanish era. In those days people weren't so educated and were still very superstitious, and they really believed this place was haunted, so no one went there. But your grandfather was someone who never believed in superstitions. He needed a home; no one else was there, and it was free. Most of his education was self-taught, and even that early on he could appreciate that building. It wasn't just a decaying structure; it was original Spanish construction with coral rock built on a vantage point to keep a lookout for possible invaders. To him, that was a castle. It was his castle. He was even the one to figure out that the 'ghost lights' were simple fireflies."

Nora looked at me in amazement. "So it was all true?"

"Yes."

"Even the shark and the turtle?"

"Yes."

She rolled her eyes. "He shouldn't have done that. We were even discussing that in class the other day. Do you have any idea how endangered sea turtles are?"

At that moment I really wanted to find that teacher and slap her silly. "Does your teacher know anything about hunger? I mean real hunger? Your grandfather had nothing at that time. Absolutely nothing! He was living day to day. Do you know how grandiose a meal that was for him to still remember it almost fifty years later? That would have been the most he had eaten in a year!"

And as I was telling her this, it started to dawn on me. "Your grandfather had a very hard life. As bad as it was, I never heard him tell one sad story. He always talked about the shark he got, but he never complained about all the fish that got away. He didn't make up stories; he told them the way he saw them—not to protect us, but he just really believed in the positive." I surprised myself, I think, as much as I did Nora. I had never seen it in that light until I had to explain it to her.

So instead of having my daughter visit and not know what to say, I found something that she had in common with my Dad, and the future generation ended up preserving the past one. We have to teach our children that the Alzheimer's patient sitting in front of us wasn't always like this. Once upon a time, he was young and had adventures that could surprise us. It's hard to see the frail, elderly individual as anything other than an Alzheimer's patient. But somewhere in there is the person we remember. Sometimes it's hard to see that, and sometimes we're blinded by it.

Chapter 12

Family Outings

I felt horrible after having to leave my dad at an ALF. At first, the hardest part was not being able to take him out anywhere. If we were to take him to the corner for coffee, he would assume we were taking him back home. It would be a disaster when he realized that he was going back to the ALF. I suffered guilt every time I left. I called him every day, and all he would do was ask when he was coming home and then reprimand me for how uncaring we were for having left him. But after a while a funny thing happened: he settled in. He made friends at the ALF and began to enjoy living in a house where he wasn't criticized for his odd behavior. He liked living in a house with other men who shared his interests. I think I was happier than he was when I finally decided I could take him out for lunch. But that turned out to be a disaster too.

Family outings can be complicated when someone has Alzheimer's. Our Germans walk at a slower pace and have difficulty moving. Someone always needs to watch them to make sure they don't wander off. They may forget the people they are with, start talking to themselves, or interact with others in a manner that may embarrass you.

With all these possible risks, why go out? Because no one wants to stay inside the same four walls all day, every day. If your German is in a nursing home or an ALF, chances are you will only see him once a week. A visit spent just sitting around for an hour isn't really pleasant for anyone. It makes many people think of visiting with the old and sick, of hospital care and other sad things. Taking the German out for a few hours offers so much more stimulation for everyone. Eventually your family will start to associate visits with happy experiences.

When we visited my father, we would first take him to lunch and then go someplace else, like the park or a store. A family outing doesn't have to be a big event; you can simply take the German with you to do your grocery shopping. It's just about spending time together.

Whenever Nora came along on a visit, she always wanted to eat junk food. If we took Dad to lunch with my sister and her kids (all six of them), we wanted a fast meal. On the days that it was just my father and me, I liked to go to a nice sit-down restaurant. One time I thought he would enjoy going to Denny's. They have a senior special; it was near the ALF; and no one there spoke Spanish. If he started saying silly things, no one would understand him.

We sat in a nice booth. He liked the booth. I showed him the menu with all the pictures, explaining what dishes each picture showed. Dad was very pleased that he got to choose his own lunch. He knew how to say "thank you" in English, so every time the waitress brought something out he said proudly, "Thank you."

I was happy; he was happy . . . and then the bill came. He didn't say "thank you" then. "Moraima, don't pay it! That woman didn't bring me my meal!" he yelled, pointing at the waitress. The waitress didn't speak Spanish, but she was caught off guard.

"Did he just call me a name?"

"Oh, no, no. Please understand. My father has Alzheimer's. He doesn't remember that you brought him his lunch."

"Don't pay her! She has to bring me my food first!" Everyone in the restaurant was looking at us. Since no one spoke Spanish, they thought Dad was insulting the waitress.

The waitress leaned over and showed my father the empty plate in front of him. "This . . . your . . . plate. You . . . already . . . ate."

At least she made an effort to understand. My dad just looked at her, confused. "You bring me an empty plate? Here I am starving and you have the nerve to mock me!"

I told the waitress, "Just bring him another plate and charge me for it."

While we were waiting, I noticed all the other patrons giving us dirty looks. Apparently everyone liked this waitress. Pretty soon she came out with the second plate and another bill. She smiled at my dad and made sure he saw her putting the plate down. "We . . . good . . . now?"

Dad nodded his head and said to me, "You can pay her now." Then he turned to the waitress and said, "Thank you." Of course I gave her a big tip. I waited for Dad to finish eating, but he didn't take one bite. "You know, I'm not really hungry anymore." Well, of course not; he had already gorged himself the first time around!

I turned to call the waitress back. "Excuse me, miss . . ." Immediately the entire restaurant fell silent. Absolutely everyone was looking at us.

The waitress came back, still smiling. "What now, hon?" And everyone watched, waiting to see what I would say. "Can I just have a little box . . . please?"

"Sure, no problem."

I just sat there looking straight ahead to avoid making eye contact with any of the other patrons. It was still very quiet. The waitress came back with the box. I packed the food, and we got out of there. By the time I got to the car I was sweating bullets. Dad sat next to me with his box of second helpings. "Well, they were nice. We should come back here next week." Over my dead body! That was the last time I would take him any place where no one spoke Spanish.

As you can see, some complications from Alzheimer's are caused not by the disease itself but by other people's reactions to the symptoms. No one in that restaurant really did anything wrong. They heard someone getting loud and interpreted Dad's behavior as hostility toward their favorite waitress. Their reactions didn't affect my father, but they made me extremely nervous. There's always a risk of embarrassment when you go out with an Alzheimer's patient. But embarrassment is temporary. And outings are far more enjoyable than sitting in a room doing nothing, checking your watch to see when the hour is up. Of course I do recommend taking precautions against embarrassing situations. At least I tried to take precautions.

By nature, Cubans speak a little louder than most people. I figured if I took Dad to a Latin restaurant, he could get loud, and it wouldn't be such a big deal like it was at Denny's. The next time, we went to a typical Latin restaurant. Outside there was a little window for people who just wanted to get Cuban coffee or cigarettes. Inside was the main restaurant. We sat down; there was music and lots of people were talking loudly. Perfect.

Dad was very pleased because they had his favorite dish, flaming ox tail. I ordered him soup instead. While we were waiting for the food, I got a call from the hospital. I stepped aside to take care of the call. Less than two minutes later, I looked over and Dad was gone. I looked right and left trying to figure out where he had gone. All of a sudden I heard someone yelling, "Hey, this isn't Cuba! You have to pay for that!" There was a commotion at the outside coffee shop. "Hey, get back here! Come back!" I then saw my dad walk triumphantly through the door holding a pack of cigarettes.

"Dad, what did you do?"

"Oh, I went and got cigarettes."

Then I saw a man rushing in after Dad. "Hey, this man didn't pay for that. You know him?"

I fought the temptation to say no and walk away. "Yes, he's with me."

"Listen, he didn't pay for those cigarettes."

"I know. Here." I gave the guy a ten and let him keep the change.

My dad looked at the guy and said, "See, I told you she would pay. My daughter is a doctor; she will come back later and pay."

"Dad, how come you never forget that I'm going to come later and pay for all these things?" And he just gave me a tricky little smile, which made me wonder if he wasn't faking his Alzheimer's to some degree. But that was wishful thinking.

We sat down again and the waitress brought the soup (luckily he had forgotten the ox tail). Then I noticed him staring at the bowl. There was a little black speck in the middle of the soup, a little piece of burnt onion. I thought, *Let me nip this in the bud before it becomes another incident.* "Oh, here, let me just remove that."

"Don't touch it!" My father yelled in a deep, commanding voice. "Do not remove it from there." He called to the waitress, "Miss, come back here."

She came over. "Yes, what is it?"

"Do you see that?"

She looked at it. "Oh, yeah, but that's part of the soup." I looked at her in despair and raised my eyebrows.

I took my spoon. "Dad, it's nothing. Let me just remove it."

"Don't you touch that! Don't you realize this soup is poisoned?"

Oh, no. His paranoia was acting up. My heart went down to my toes. It sank past the toes, past the shoes, past the floor. "Dad, Dad, look, the soup is not poisoned. I'm going to have a sip and . . ."

"Don't! I'm not going to let my daughter poison herself!" He turned to the waitress, "Would you drink this soup?" The waitress looked at me and must have realized that I was horrified and trying to apologize without saying the words. And she was very nice and tolerant and said, "Gramps, I'll show you. I'll eat some of your soup and you'll see it's not poisoned. Now if I eat some of your soup will you eat the rest?"

"Yes, but you have to drink it first." So she took his spoon, scooped up the part of the soup with the burnt onion and slurped it all down.

"See! It's not poisoned."

"OK, I believe you. Now get me another spoon because you slobbered all over mine."

Oh, Lord have mercy! And the waitress looked at me, put her hand on my shoulder and said, "Don't worry, my mother does this to me all the time." I'll bet that waitress still remembers me because I gave her the biggest tip that anyone in that restaurant had ever given.

You read about "memory loss," and you think that means misplacing keys. You never expect memory loss to manifest itself in such unpredictable ways. Forgetting a meal and causing a scene in a restaurant is not something that you generally expect. But those are the little "fun" moments that catch you off guard. My dad was not doing these things on purpose to embarrass me; his brain simply did not function properly anymore. To believe that these actions were deliberate is to believe theft is a symptom of Alzheimer's. Obviously it isn't. But Alzheimer's patients will go to the store to pick up milk or socks. They'll pick up what they need and then forget and walk out without paying. They didn't go into the store with the intention of stealing, but the security guard might not view it that way. There's that human factor again. It's very easy to read a list of symptoms, but it's very different when they manifest themselves in real life. Perhaps I should have just followed my daughter's fast food plan and avoided taking Dad to sit-down restaurants.

Of course Nora generally wanted fast food because she was in a rush to end the visit. As she got older it became increasingly difficult to make her visit her grandfather. So I did what any good parent would do. I tricked her. We were already driving in the car when she noticed. "Hey, this isn't the way to the mall."

"Well, I thought we could visit your grandpa first."

"What? We'll be there all day!"

"Not necessarily. We can take him to the mall with us."

She rolled her eyes, crossed her arms, and stared out the car window. It wasn't that she hated him or even claimed to anymore, but visiting Dad still upset her. Dad didn't remember who Nora was, and I think that she felt her grandfather had abandoned her. I also think the absence of her grandfather was particularly difficult for Nora because he was the only father figure she had in her life up to that point. When she was really young she even had called him Papa until he corrected her.

Dad's response to our arrival at the ALF didn't help. I announced, "Look, Pop, Nora came with me today."

Dad looked at her sideways. "That's not Nora." Nora didn't do or say anything; she just sighed. Trying to make it up to her; I decided we should just head straight to the mall. Unfortunately Nora had to take the backseat so that I could converse with Dad and keep him focused. Nora wasn't saying anything, so I tried to include her. I asked for her input on some random thing I was discussing with Dad. Before she could answer, Dad turned around, looking for Nora. Keep in mind that for Alzheimer's patients, out of sight can mean out of mind. Dad wasn't interacting with Nora and didn't see her in the backseat, so he forgot there was someone else in the car. "Where's Nora? How did the neighbor's kid get here?" Nora remained silent for the rest of the drive.

As awkward as the situation was, I tried to stay positive. I took them both to my favorite store, where I saw a gorgeous dress suit. "Nora, look at this! I just love it! Oh, they even have one in your size! We can be like . . ." When I turned to show her, she was already gone. "Well, I guess it's just you and me, Pop. How about we go to the men's section and get you a new . . . Oh my God, they're having a sale on shoes!" While I paused to look at a pretty pair of flats, he disappeared too. Now I had a problem.

I rushed out in time to see him following a teenage couple that had just left the store. I came up behind him just in time to hear him say to the girl, "Your tits are so big you are going to fall forward." You can imagine my embarrassment. The teenagers' reactions were anything but pretty.

The young boyfriend verbally and most adamantly defended his lady's honor. His lady chimed in with her own remarks. Not one to take insults well, Dad returned their foul language with some of his own. Their comments are not suitable to be repeated, but trust me, it got nasty. The crowd that gathered didn't help either. Some of the onlookers started taking sides. The younger people said my dad was a pervert, and the more mature group asserted that the teenagers were a pair of ignorant, angry punks. Oh dear Lord, Dad had started another riot!

Dad had always been respectful to women. It was not his intention to insult this girl and start a fight with her boyfriend. But common sense and logic (and that little voice that tells us to keep our thoughts to ourselves) start shutting down as Alzheimer's progresses. As a result, a German doesn't hesitate to point out anything he finds interesting or offensive about anyone. It doesn't matter if it's a muscle-bound boxer or a busty teenager.

The insults and threats toward my father from said busty teenage girl's boyfriend (as well as the crowd) got to a point where I had to physically stand between Dad and the couple to protect Dad while profusely apologizing for him. The couple really didn't seem to understand the term "Alzheimer's."

As the people in the crowd started bickering among themselves, I tried to push Dad out of the group. Of course I had to keep turning around to calm down the angry boyfriend and reassure him that he had won the fight. He could now proudly go home after out-shouting a senile old man. When I turned around, wouldn't you know it, Dad had vanished again!

There was only one direction he could have gone. I went to find Nora first, which was easy since she only went to four stores in the entire mall. Sure enough, she was in the music shop. "Sorry, sweetie, but your grandpa wandered off. Please help me find him." We both went looking and found him almost at the end of the mall, totally unaware of the commotion he had created (or the amount of stress he had caused me).

He looked at me and said, "Did you get lost? I've been looking for you."

"Good," said Nora, "you found him. If you need me, I'll be back at the music store."

"Actually, Nora, we need to go home now."

"But we just got here."

"I know. I'm sorry, but Grandpa may have created a riot at the other end of the mall, and we really need to get out of here."

Disheartened, Nora looked at me and said, "Again?"

Yes, we had some fun family outings. A lot of people would say, "Why risk it?" When you go on these outings, you'll pray for an uneventful day and rejoice if your dad doesn't try to take his clothes off in the store. But afterward, when it's all over, you're not going to remember the quiet, uneventful outings. When you think back, you'll remember the time you were chased out the restaurant by an angry group of truckers. Those are the moments that stick with you: the ones you can laugh at long after they pass.

Chapter 13

Other People and Other Experiences

The best laid plans of . . . well, you know the rest. It's very easy to read instructions or listen to advice and work out the perfect plan. There is no such thing as a perfect plan. The thing that most people forget when making these plans is other people. When you are dealing with a relative with Alzheimer's, you want the whole family to work together. There is a chance that you have one or more people in your family who, for better or worse, will have an uncalculated impact on your plans. Let's call them the X factors.

The Naysayer

The naysayer has difficulty understanding the nature of Alzheimer's. They say, "Oh, it's not Alzheimer's" or "That's not a real disease" or "It's not that serious." My mother, for all her strength, could not accept that my father's forgetfulness meant he was sick. Perhaps you have a relative who struggles with the concept of Alzheimer's as a disease, particularly if they're from the old-school mentality. Dad already had schizophrenia; he couldn't have two illnesses. The reality was that my mom couldn't handle Dad's diagnosis, so she went into denial. That's not uncommon. Denial is generally our first reaction to bad news. Some folks will leave the doctor's diploma-encrusted office angrily saying "she's a quack," "someone made a mistake," and, of course, "let's just forget what she said." Then they'll go home and act normal and try to ignore the little things until something happens that's so big it forces them to recognize the truth.

The Outsider

The outsider is not immediately associated with the family through blood or marriage but is still involved in caring for the German. Outsiders include a boyfriend or girlfriend, a close friend, a coworker, or the German's caretaker. A tug of war for attention can put a strain on your relationships with the outsider and the German. A new boyfriend might be less than thrilled if you cancel a date for a doctor's appointment. I know my boss and some of my coworkers didn't appreciate when I had to take off in the middle of the day because Dad had wandered off. They may have difficulty understanding because they haven't stood in your place; they're on the outside looking in. The thing to do is to explain the situation and hope that they understand. Likewise, when others care enough to help you with the German, sharing responsibilities can bring you closer. This is why caretakers will sometimes feel like part of the family. Let's say your boyfriend goes with you to look for your German instead of getting upset over a missed movie date. When you have friends like that, make sure you show your appreciation.

The Con Man

People outside or inside the family can take advantage of your German's affliction for their own gain. The con man (or woman) might trick your loved one into signing over checks or giving up personal things. Alzheimer's patients will not remember if they lent money to someone the day before, and a con man might show up every day to borrow money. Some of these individuals may be either very smooth or very intimidating. A con man can be polite and reassuring, and even if you notice something wrong like missing money or physical injury to your German, the con man will still say that everything is fine. Some people who have an immediate relationship to the German may use that connection to manipulate the rest of the family. If you are faced with a con man, separate them; cut off all ties between them and the German and possibly your whole family. If the con man persists, you might have to get the authorities involved.

The Real Estate Agent

Real estate agents want to send their Germans out to a home when it isn't really necessary or want to keep them near when they really need to go. These people are making choices for emotional and personal reasons. If there is any doubt about where a patient should stay, the best recourse is to get an outside opinion from the doctor.

The Incredible Helper

No matter the situation, these people always offer their help. For me, the incredible helper was my boyfriend. He was an outside influence who, for some reason, Dad would listen to. Perhaps Robert reminded Dad of a friend, or maybe after forty years of living with women, Dad was just happy to have another guy around. I don't know. But I could count on Robert to come and talk my dad into doing what he needed to do. Be careful not to become too dependent on incredible helpers because they might feel you're taking advantage of them, and a day may come when they'll have to leave.

Apart from big tips and angry teenagers, there are other expenses that come with Alzheimer's, things you would never think to consider. One day while visiting Dad, I noticed that he was talking funny. He wasn't wearing his dentures. I went to get his dentures, but they weren't by his bed. I asked him. Of course he didn't know. Neither did the staff, but the staff did assure me that it would find the dentures.

I called during the week, and they hadn't found Dad's dentures. "Dr. Trujillo, I looked everywhere, even in the grass, inch by inch. I couldn't find them anywhere." During this time my dad was eating puree. By the next Saturday I went back, hoping that they had found his teeth. When I got there, they gave me a bill. Turns out there had been some trouble with one of the toilets that got so bad they had to call a plumber. At least they found the dentures. My dad, however, was not so thrilled about the find. "I'm not putting those in my mouth! They were in the toilet!"

"But I cleaned them," insisted the staff member. "I cleaned them very thoroughly."

"I don't care! They were at the bottom of the toilet with everyone's crap! I'm not putting everyone's crap in my mouth!"

Great, now I had to get him a new set of dentures. In all honesty, I wouldn't have put those in my mouth either. So I made an appointment with the dentist, and they took care of everything except the bill. Dad's insurance no longer covered him for replacement dentures. So not only did I have to pay for the dentures out of pocket, but I also had to pay the ALF's plumbing bill. I couldn't visit my father the next weekend because I had to cover some extra shifts to help pay the bills. The weekend after that, the new dentures were ready. I took Dad to try them on, and they fit like a glove. All's well that ends well. The day after we got him his new dentures I got a call from the ALF.

"He doesn't want to wear them."

"What? Why?"

"He thinks they're the ones that fell in the toilet."

In the background I could hear my dad screaming, "Those are the ones that fell in the toilet. I saw them." He got on the phone, and I tried to correct him.

"No, Dad, remember that I took you to the dentist? We threw away the other teeth."

"No, I threw them away. You are trying to trick me. There was no dentist. I remember flushing the toilet, and when I looked down, the teeth fell in."

"Then you knew this whole time where they were! You said you didn't know where they were!"

"You see? You are trying to trick me!"

"Ah, Pops, why couldn't you forget the toilet and remember the dentist?"

It had to be Murphy's Law. I had expected something to go wrong because at the time I was trying to arrange a special meeting. I had been dating someone for a while, and I wanted to introduce him to Dad. I wanted everything to be perfect, so of course something had to go wrong.

I invited the whole family to a late lunch at a nice sit-down restaurant. Since Dad refused to wear his teeth, I thought that some soup and spaghetti that wouldn't require much chewing would be good. So we went to this little Italian place in Hialeah. My whole family liked it because not only did they have great pastas, but they also had pizza.

With something for everyone, we were having a delightful time. I sat Dad in front of my boyfriend, and after everyone had ordered I said, "Dad, this is Robert. He is my boyfriend." It's difficult enough introducing a new love interest to the family; I didn't know what to expect now that Alzheimer's was a factor. Robert gave Dad a firm handshake and introduced himself. I held my breath as Dad looked Robert over.

"You're bald."

"I noticed," replied Robert.

"I can fix that. All you have to do is rub some garlic on your head and that will make the hair grow . . ." and he kept going. Oh, Dad, why did you have to make comments about his bald head? It can be awkward when someone with Alzheimer's goes off into his own world and starts a rambling conversation that isn't necessarily related to anything anyone else is talking about. But just as I thought I was heading toward a breakup, not only did Robert not get offended by the various far-flung treatments for baldness my father was ranting on about, but he also played along. That's the correct thing to do when a German starts displaying this behavior.

But by now you probably know what I'm going to say. Don't interrupt them; don't correct them; don't get upset. Think as if you are talking to a young toddler. Preschoolers have a tendency to ramble on about nonsensical things. Since they're just learning to talk, parents don't generally stop them; they just smile and encourage their children to continue. Same thing with Alzheimer's patients. Smile as they talk. Say a few things in agreement not because you really agree but to show that you are there. Hold their hand or put an arm around them. You are demonstrating to them a connection. These gestures show that you are there, that you are listening, and that you are happy. And that makes them happy, even if they can only show it by continuing to ramble.

I didn't have to explain any of this to Robert. He automatically knew how to act. No matter what comment Dad made, Robert ran with it. The two of them hit it off like old friends. Robert was even calling him "Old Man" within the first fifteen minutes. The waitress brought the food, and

Dad began to eat his spaghetti. He looked down at his waist and suddenly said, "Excuse me, Robert; I have to go get my belt."

"Old Man, where are you going?"

"I'm just going outside to get my belt."

"The only thing outside is the car." I said. "Your closet is back at the home, half an hour away."

"My belt is outside and I'm going to get it."

"But, Grandpa," Nora spoke up, "you're wearing your belt."

My father looked down. "This!" When I heard him raise his voice I thought, *Oh no.* He took the belt off, stood up, and announced to the entire restaurant, "This is not my belt!" Robert, Nora, everyone at the table—even my godmother was with us that day—were all telling him, "That is your belt. Put it back on." And Dad persisted. "This is not my belt! It is an imposter belt."

I kept telling the rest of them to stop contradicting him. Then I turned to Dad and realized his pants were falling off. I remembered the only time my dad had taken his belt to my butt. Now it felt like I was being belted again—with humiliation. "Pop, I know it's not your belt, but why don't you just wear it for now?"

"I do not wear other men's clothes! Now, I am going outside to get my belt!" And his pants kept sliding down.

"No, Dad, sit down! You're right; it's the wrong belt. Here, let me take care of that." I took the belt and walked outside. After five minutes I came back. "Here it is; I found your belt." Before he could look at it, I put it on his pants and buckled it up. "There, all taken care of." I went back to my seat and started eating.

Dad examined the belt. He looked at me the same way he used to when I was seven and had done something wrong. "You think I'm an idiot? This is the same belt!"

Fortunately we didn't have to cut the trip short to go back for his belt. The restaurant was in the same shopping center as a Kmart. Robert and I took Dad, who entered the store with dignity, holding his pants up. It turned out he was willing to settle for a brand new belt. He tried it on, liked it, and let me pay for it. That's when Robert asked me, "Are you sure he didn't just want a new belt?"

There is one more person who you don't always expect to be a factor: the clown. In my case, that role was played by my boyfriend. Germans are easily influenced. If they hear or see something, they'll focus all their attention on that new stimulus. My boyfriend took advantage of this.

Robert and I had been going together for a while. He met all the criteria of a good boyfriend: my daughter liked him; he would come when I had an emergency; and my mother didn't chase him away with a broomstick. After some time, he started getting comfortable around us.

Dad still couldn't remember Nora clearly and it upset her. Since Nora didn't always want to visit her grandfather, Robert would sometimes accompany me. One day we took Dad to the supermarket. I had just found a parking space when an old man cut me off and took it. Dad got upset. "Hey, he had no right to that spot. You had the indicators on."

"Dad, calm down. It's no big deal. Look, there's another space right over there."

We parked and got out, but all of a sudden Robert started pointing, "Old Man, there! That's the guy who took our parking space."

Dad huffed. "Who does he think he is? Hey, you! Yeah, you! That was our parking space!"

Robert egged him on. "Yeah, let's go over there and teach him a lesson." *Oh, my God,* I thought. *I'm dating a crazy person.*

As Dad and Robert went to confront the old man I grabbed Robert by the back of his shirt. "What are you doing?"

"Oh, calm down, China, we're not really going to fight him." I pointed at my dad, who was already yelling in the other old man's face. And I heard Robert laughing under his smile, "Well, he did steal our parking space. We have to scare him a little." Then he turned to the fighting seniors and yelled, "Yeah, Old Man, you tell him!" Robert started to walk away, and I pulled him back again. *"What* are you doing?"

"It's two on one; that old geezer is going to back down and leave. Don't worry." As he joined my dad in this screaming contest, the old man didn't back down. He became more aggressive. Everyone was starting to stare. The old man was the smartest of the three because he eventually did turn and walk away. *Oh good, it's over.*

"That's right, you old bastard, walk away like a coward!" *Robert! What the hell are you doing?* Just like that, the old man turned around and got back in their faces louder than before.

I would have been better off with the cranky preteen than these two toddlers. Fine, if they were going to act like children, I was going to treat them like children. "If you're going to fight, I'm leaving! And I'm leaving you both!" I was dead serious; I hate being embarrassed in public. Dad saw me turn back to the car. "Robert," I heard him say, "I think she's really leaving."

"No, no, she's just going to sit in the car."

Then they saw that I was actually driving away. In the rearview mirror I saw them running after me. Afraid that if I left them behind the cops might arrest them, I stopped the car long enough for them to get in. At least I taught them both a lesson.

"We showed him, didn't we, Old Man?"

Apparently they didn't learn the lesson.

"Can you believe that guy?"

"I can't believe you!" I exclaimed. "Didn't you notice I almost left you back there because of your stupidity? You guys were about to start a fight over a parking space!"

"That was our space," my dad said.

"You said it, Old Man. That guy's gonna think twice before he steals someone else's parking space."

I glared at Robert in a manner that conveyed the message: *Damn it, Robert, shut up! Just let him forget it.* I think he understood.

"Of course, we had to leave for China's sake."

"Oh, yes, women should not be around fights."

At the end of the visit Robert had to answer to me. "What the hell were you doing?" I asked.

"Now, baby, let me explain . . . it's a guy thing; you wouldn't understand."

"Try me."

"Your dad is a man."

"I noticed that."

"No, I mean he has to establish his manhood. Your family is all girls. And in the home he just sits there. But what you saw—that's a man opportunity. That was a chance for him to show how tough he was and feel like a real man."

"So starting fights with total strangers, acting like a complete jackass, and almost having the cops called on you is a man opportunity?"

"Exactly! I did it for him. And you can't tell me that he wasn't happier about getting into a fight than when you took him to the mall last week."

Technically, he was right. Dad did get a boost in pride as well as stimulation from the borderline barbaric situation, which Robert was tactlessly trying to portray as a brilliant plan he had created to better my father's mental health. Dad did feel manlier for some time after that. But just because Robert was right didn't mean I was going to acknowledge that. It also didn't mean I wasn't going to make him suffer for it. That's an angry girlfriend thing; he wouldn't understand.

The Really BIG Incident

It was midafternoon when I got the call. An ALF employee asked, "I'm sorry, Dr. Trujillo, but by any chance did you take your father out today?"

"No, is he missing?"

"Yes. I'm sorry, we can't find him anywhere."

Knowing that my father liked to go to the supermarket café every Saturday for coffee and cigarettes, I asked if they had checked there.

"Yes, but he wasn't there either. He just wandered off!"

Even after all the times my father had wandered off, it still made me uneasy. But it was important to stay calm. We had found him every time. Sometimes he had even found a phone and called me. He couldn't have gotten that far.

I switched into bounty hunter mode. Unfortunately, that day there was a massive demonstration all down 40th Street, so the road was closed. There were protesters everywhere. But I was determined to get there. I took all the side streets and got to the little grocery store where Dad spent his Saturdays. He had to be close. Logically he would be in the perimeter between the supermarket plaza and the ALF. Maybe he took the wrong street back and that confused him. Perhaps he saw someone or something that caught his attention and he followed that. All the while people in buses drove down the street honking, yelling, and waving flags. So, I stood by the supermarket and tried to think what could have caught his attention. I drove up and down the streets looking for him. Suddenly, my cell phone rang. I thought, *Oh, good, that's him now.* But instead it was my aunt. "Moraima! Moraima, are you sitting down?"

"What happened?"

"Are you anywhere where you can watch television?"

"No."

"Your father is on television!"

167

"What? Where?"

"He's at the Orange Bowl. He's marching with the protesters. He's got a Cuban hat and a flag, and he's screaming 'Viva Cuba Libre!'"

You have got to be kidding me. The Orange Bowl? How the hell did he get down there? To give you a visual, the Orange Bowl (the former football home of the championship-winning Dolphins) was over twenty miles from the ALF. "Auntie C, you're closer than I am. Do you think you can find him and take him to your house?"

"They aren't letting anyone drive into the area."

"Please, Auntie, we've been looking for him for hours."

"OK . . . I'll try."

Good. I hung up with her, called Robert, and asked him to go with me to pick up my dad. On the way, my aunt called and said she had him.

"He's here at my house with me and my daughter. But he is not a happy camper. We're trying to keep him from leaving, but Moraima, he is scaring me. I just hid all the knives because he's talking about starting a political revolution and conquering the world. He is *really* out of it."

Robert and I knew to we had to walk in there like nothing was going on. It was just a casual Saturday family get-together. Nothing had happened. From the moment we walked in, my aunt's eyes were as big as an owl's.

"I had to make him coffee," she said as she glared at us. "I know he's agitated and wound up already but he demanded coffee. My daughter even went to buy him cigarettes. He's in the kitchen now, smoking."

I went in the kitchen and there he was, smoking, a cup of coffee in one hand and an American flag tucked into his collar. "Hey, Pop, how are you doing?"

He started rambling—all this nonsense that he had to run because he was being persecuted and was trying to fight for the freedom of the people. He was switching from one subject to another. He repeated all the chants that he had heard in the rally as if they pertained to him. The experience was bringing up the paranoia of his schizophrenia. Finally I cut him off.

"Dad, Dad, here, drink some water." He looked dehydrated; he was badly sunburned. I said, "Here, have some water, drink some fluids, and then we have to go to the hospital."

"I am not going to any damn hospital! You think I'm crazy!"

Oh no, we had a problem. I backed off. Robert tapped me on the shoulder and addressed my father, "Hey, Trujillo, get in the car. Men ride in the front."

"Yes, my brother, let's take the fight to them." He showed Robert a lot of man-to-man respect, shaking his hand and actually doing what Robert said. And at that point, he had only met Robert a few times. Men!

Halfway down the road, my dad looked at Robert. "You're tricking me into taking me to the hospital."

"Well, look, I want to make sure the doctor looks you over before we go start the revolution."

"All right, all right, trick me. That's OK." And he continued talking nonsense.

When we got to the hospital the doctor asked for my dad's history, but Dad kept giving him the wrong information.

The only thing he stated accurately was his date of birth. When they asked him about his medical problems he said, "None."

"Any medications?"

"None. Have you ever met a man that needed medications?"

And it just kept getting worse. When an intern came with a wheelchair and asked Dad to sit, my father looked at him and very considerately warned him, "Do you want me to answer you now or later? I am a man! Men do not use wheelchairs! Men do not need medicines! Men do not belong in hospitals!" While that young intern pondered his career choice, I tried to give the nurse Dad's real information. Dad didn't like this and got mad at me—I mean really irate. It soon became very clear to everyone in the ER that Dad needed to be admitted to the psychiatric ward. They called an orderly to take over for the intern, who had mysteriously disappeared, but Dad still refused to cooperate. He didn't care that this orderly had at least 150 pounds on him. Better said, Alzheimer's refused to let him process this fact. He was ready to face off against this rather large orderly just as he had against the inexperienced intern.

Robert went to the doctor. "Look, he needs to be admitted."

"I know," said the doctor. "Why don't you take him to the side, and when we're ready to—"

"You're not taking me anywhere!" screamed Dad. "I'm leaving."

Dad made a beeline for the door. He wasn't even running; he was just walking out. I kept pleading with him. He flat-out refused to listen to me. Robert stepped in again. "Hey, Trujillo, you and me are going this way."

"OK."

That's it? No fighting? No lecturing? Forget that I'm your daughter, the one who's always taken you to the doctor before. I'm the one who actually studied medicine and spent the last half hour explaining to you why you should stay in the hospital. Oh, just forget all that and listen to a guy you've only met three times! I know I should have been grateful that the situation was resolved that easily, but come on!

And my dad actually followed Robert into the elevator. Robert went with him to the fourth floor (the psychiatric ward), walked him in, and finally convinced him to stay. "OK, Trujillo, I'll see you tomorrow."

My dad looked at Robert. "Don't forget to bring me some cigarettes."

Chapter 14

It Gets Worse

The frustration I felt toward Robert helped me understand the anger my mother must have felt toward my dad. After we initially put my dad in the ALF, my mother had a moment of independent awakening. With her own savings, she bought a house in a new development. After the Orange Bowl incident, she recanted her decision about putting Dad in a home. Even if her decision had been necessary at the time, none of us were happy with it. My mother never talked about her feelings; she never even let anyone mention "the home" in our home. I can only assume that she experienced guilt that climaxed with Dad's latest wandering misadventure. I guess she thought that since she no longer had to look after me or Nora, she would be free to give my father the proper attention he needed. Everyone was thrilled that Grandpa was coming back to the family. Dad, of course, had another opinion.

Mistakes were made.

Mom converted the extra bedroom in her house into Dad's new room—she still had not forgiven him for the hooker episode. And it was probably wise for them to sleep separately and avoid another such incident. Fortunately, I was now far enough away that I didn't have to deal with their old-married-couple bickering . . . or so I thought.

As will happen to everyone, especially older people, Dad got sick. He was diagnosed with COPD (chronic obstruction pulmonary disease). The doctor gave him a pill and told him to take one every day to treat his shortness of breath. As my father's caretaker, my mother made the same mistakes as before and trusted him to take his own pills. Trouble was that he had Alzheimer's, so he forgot to take his medication. In the middle of the night he woke her up because he couldn't breathe. He asked her to give him his pill. Half-asleep, she went to the kitchen, got the pill, fixed a glass of water, swallowed the pill, washed it down with the water, and went back to bed. As she was about to turn the lamp off, my wheezing father asked, "Woman . . . *gasp* . . . where's . . . *gasp* . . . my . . . *gasp* . . . pill?" And that woke her up.

At three in the morning, I was awoken by my mother's phone call. She was hysterical. "I took your father's pill! I took your father's pill! I've been poisoned!" In the background I could hear, "My pill! *Gasp*. Give me . . . *gasp* . . . my pill! *Gasp*. I'm dying, woman! *Gasp*."

"Mom, give him the pill!"

"That's what I was doing, but I was sleepy! He woke me up! I had a pill and a glass; it was a reflex!"

"You are not going to die! Give him another pill!"

To make sure that neither one of them would die, I drove all the way to her house very early in the morning. *Unbelievable,* I thought. *I'm a zip code away, and I still have to deal with their late-night incidents.* My father finally did take his medication, but he couldn't go to sleep because my mother was having a fit. She was convinced that she had poisoned herself. I stayed with them to calm her down and assure her that nothing was going to happen. Finally, at six a.m., they went to bed. I had barely enough time to go home and get ready for work.

There were other incidents, most of which my mother didn't tell me about. But the one where the house caught fire . . . that one I found out about first. After years of worrying that my father would accidentally burn the house down, it was my mother who got the flames going. After cooking, she was cleaning the stove with a towel. The towel started to smolder, so she shook it to put out the embers. In the process, the curtains caught fire.

I got a call. "Moraima, the house is on fire!"

"Oh, my God! Are you OK?"

"No, my house is on fire!"

"What happened? What did the firefighters say?"

"What firefighters?"

"You didn't call the fire department?"

"No, I'm calling you!"

Then a sickening reality dawned on me. "Are you still inside the house?"

"Yes!"

"Mom, hang up! Call 911! Get Dad and get out of the house!"

I hung up, panicked that she might try to call me again, drove down there, and thank God, the firefighters were already there. It wasn't the big, all-consuming fire that I had imagined. It was a minor kitchen roast. All her neighbors were out in the street watching. I saw my mother crying hysterically to one of the firefighters. "You don't understand! He has arteriosclerosis!"

"Mom, what happened?"

"They won't let me go back in. I couldn't find your father. He's still in there!"

I started thinking, *Oh my God, the smoke got him!* Then one of the firefighters came out. "Ma'am, we checked. There is no one in there."

My mother cried out, "Oh, I knew it! He's already dead!"

"No, ma'am, we checked twice! There is no sign of anyone in there. Are you sure he didn't walk out before you did?"

"No, no, he's dead! I know he is!"

Suddenly, I felt a pat on my arm. It was the neighbor's kid. "Hey, isn't that the guy they're looking for?"

Sure enough, across the street sitting on the pavement, comfortably leaning back on the sidewalk directly in front of my mother's house was my dad. He looked fine, but I went over to check. "Dad, are you OK? Are you hurt?"

My father looked up at me. "How stupid do you think I am? I saw smoke and instead of calling 911, she started talking to you. When I saw that, I just walked out and saved myself."

"And you left Mom inside?"

"That woman is crazy! China, take me back to the home before she kills me."

The moral of this story is that just because you have Alzheimer's doesn't mean you will lose all your preservation instincts.

After the firefighters left, we inspected the house. The fire damage was minimal and confined to the kitchen. My mother didn't appreciate being called "the crazy one" by the person she considered "the sick one." Her options were to place him in a new home or become a better supervisor, spending every waking moment watching over Dad.

"Take me back to the home!" Dad shouted as I was explaining this to Mom.

"What? You call me crazy! You set my house on fire! And now you want to leave?"

"You see, China, you see! I told you she was crazy! I know she started the fire!"

"You distracted me!"

"I wasn't even in the room! That's how crazy you are!"

"Dad, Mom, please—"

"I'm crazy? Fine! You want to leave? Then leave! I'm kicking you out! And don't think for a minute that I'll take you back!"

"Promise?"

Oh brother, I couldn't get a word in edgewise. Dad stormed off to his room. I picked up the phone by the charred wall to call Dad's ALF and see if they would take him back. The girl there was very happy; she hadn't heard from me in a while. Then Mom realized who I was talking to. "You're not calling those incompetents that lost him?" On her end the girl heard this and I picked up a tremor of fear in her voice. "Oh no, it's her, isn't it?"

"Don't you dare put your father back in that pigsty! If he goes there I'm sending the cops and I'm getting a lawyer! I will bring Channel Seven News with me . . ."

And from the phone I heard, "I'm sorry, Dr. Trujillo, we have no rooms available." Then she hung up on me.

I managed to stop my mom's ranting to ask her, "When you took Dad out of the home, what did you say to them?"

She calmed down and put on her little angelic face that only came out when she had done something terrible. "Nothing. I just pointed out to the young ladies that they were irresponsible." Then Dad came out with a bunch of his underwear in a plastic bag. He headed toward the door. "Trujillo, where are you going?"

"You told me to get out."

"Yes, but not right now."

Dad looked at me. "And you think I'm crazy."

So once again I set about the task of finding a new home. Just like the last time, Mom didn't like any of them. This time I skipped straight to the end and made the decision for her. The new home was farther from my house, but it was closer to my mother and sister. We balanced out a schedule to accommodate everyone's work week. Sis and her family visited on Saturdays, I went on Sundays, and Mom, who was retired, pretty much went any day she wanted. What I really liked was that this new place had special recreational options. They offered what they called the "Little School." Dad's new home was one of the first Assisted Living Facilities that was connected with a senior center. Remember how I mentioned this type of program before? It works like a day care.

The home charged me extra for enrolling Dad in "school," but it was worth it. For him to actively engage in activities instead of sitting around watching a television set that was constantly left on was a revolutionary idea for me. I adamantly believe that there should be more of these "Little Schools." Dad loved it. He was always properly supervised, and whenever he said something strange, no one called him out on it. Whenever I came to visit, he would say, "Look what I did at school this week!" just like a little kid. He would show me pictures he had drawn or something he had built or talk about the birthday party they had for so-and-so. His day-to-day clarity improved. I believe that the increased activity was stimulating his brain and increasing function.

Then I got a call from the teacher. "Mrs. Trujillo, I'm sorry to tell you that we're suspending your father from the program."

"What? Why? What happened?"

"He got into a fight with the bus driver."

As she filled me in on the details, I hit my forehead with the clipboard I had in my hands. This didn't happen to anyone else. I spent all my academic life being perfect. Never once did Dad get any complaint about me in school. And what does he do? He gets into a schoolyard fight!

That Sunday when I visited, he was all upset because he hadn't gone to the school that week. "Well, Dad, what did you expect? You can't be starting fights."

"I didn't start any fights."

I understood that he might have forgotten about the fight, so I calmly and nonaccusingly recounted the events, hoping to jog his memory. "Well, the bus driver said you called him some bad names and he told you to sit down. And you didn't. You started screaming at the bus driver that he was a sex offender . . ."

"He started it! He doesn't like me because I'm the only real man on the bus!"

"Dad, he's a thirtysomething man driving around old ladies in their seventies. He's not interested."

"Oh, yes he is. I've seen the way he looks at them, always smiling. So I had to defend them!"

There was nothing wrong with the bus driver. He was going beyond the call of duty. He wasn't just driving the old ladies around, he was interacting, complimenting them on their hair, making them feel pretty, making them smile. That's why I loved the school. The people really cared. Unfortunately, Dad mistook these harmless compliments for something more. Of course my dad screaming at the top of his lungs that this bus driver was a sexual predator could have affected his position. I don't think the driver ever expected one of his charges to have a full-out episode in that manner.

It's the loss of inhibition again. Remember, Germans will act out inappropriately and in ways they never did before. It's never a one-time thing; if you go through one incident like this, you'll inevitably go through several.

Don't get too upset. It's not all bad. One day, I went to visit Dad while he was still suspended from the school, and I saw my mother come storming out of the ALF. I went up to her. "Mom, Mom, what's wrong?"

It was obvious that she was furious. She just glared at me, inhaling deeply and squeezing her lips tight. I was sure the top of her head was going to explode, spewing smoke and molten lava. But she didn't say a word; she just walked away, got in her car, and drove off. Whatever she was going to say must have been so horrible that she dared not speak it in front of her daughter.

Still confused as to what was going on, I went in to see my father. He was sitting on the bed in his room, very happy to see me. "Pop, I just bumped into Mom outside. She seemed really upset." He started chuckling. So I asked him, "What did you say to her?"

He paused for a moment and finally said, "I don't remember . . . but it must have been bad because she was very angry when she left."

I never did find out what he told her, but the sight of my mother so furious that she couldn't even talk was very amusing. If I hadn't thought she might kill me, I would have taken a picture of her at that moment. She looked like a cartoon. As long as it only involves someone else, a German's loss of inhibitions can be hilarious!

Chapter 15

Inhibitions

Alzheimer's will cause a loss of inhibitions. My father was not someone who would normally remove his pants in public. Of course, he could have forgotten that if you take your belt off, the pants fall. The public outburst caused by that incident led me to avoid that particular restaurant for a while.

Patients with Alzheimer's dementia are often easily influenced by cues in their environment. Remember, as memories are erased, the brain, in an effort to maintain its function, focuses on immediate stimuli. Also, as the disease progresses, brain cells that control the concept of right and wrong are among those faculties destroyed. My dad's notion of right and wrong wasn't always rock-solid, particularly when it came to rules of possession as you'll see shortly.

To compensate for memory loss, Alzheimer's patients often replace a name they have forgotten with a new one they have just learned. Let's say that while watching television, your dad sees a character named Christina. That name will get fixed in his mind. If he comes across any woman whose name he can't remember, his brain will reach for the last stimulus associated with a female name. This phenomenon usually passes in a few hours or a few days.

It was another celebration. I invited the entire family to dinner in a very famous, upscale restaurant. Dad got dressed with his flaming suit. Everybody was all dressed up. Even Nora wore something other than ripped jeans. We went to this restaurant and everything was fine. Dad behaved like you would never believe he had Alzheimer's. It was one of those clear, crisp days for him. There were many of us at the table, and we all paid attention to make sure we kept up with his little things here and there. At the end, the waiter came over and handed me the check, and Dad still remembered that he had eaten.

As a rule I look over the check to make sure everything is fine. At the bottom I saw, handwritten, *$5.00 Ashtray*. Why were they charging me for an ashtray? Quietly and very diplomatically (since I was the one paying, I didn't want anyone to think I was being a cheapskate and questioning the bill), I signaled for the waiter to come over. I pointed at the ashtray charge and asked, "Why are you charging me for this?"

He leaned forward and said, "The charge is for the ashtray the gentleman took." The waiter indicated my father with his eyes.

I asked, "Dad, did you take the table's ashtray?"

Dad said, "Me? Of course not. Why would I do that? No way."

"Well, Dad, they're charging me five dollars for an ashtray that they believe you took."

And (I can only assume he meant to kill me with embarrassment) he said, "Five dollars," and pulled the ashtray out from his jacket pocket, "for this piece of plastic? This is not worth five dollars!" Loud enough for the entire restaurant to hear, he continued, "They are trying to charge my daughter five dollars for this ashtray! It is not worth it!" And he put it back on the table. I said to the waiter, "I'll pay you for the ashtray. I'll pay you for anything." I just wanted to get out of there. "Dad, you've got ashtrays at home."

"Well, you know, it was a pretty one, and this is a very nice restaurant, so I figured I'd keep it as a souvenir."

"Why didn't you tell me? I would have asked for one. They sell them at the cash register on the way out. They have a gift shop."

"I don't know. I thought it was just nicer to stick it in my pocket."

My old dad never would have done that. He had been the kind of person who, if I took something that didn't belong to me, would embarrass me in public and hit my hand as a punishment to teach me, "Thou shall not take what does not belong to you." I could not believe it. I had even more trouble believing that after I kindly, politely, diplomatically confronted him with what people said he'd done, he would pull it out of his pocket and show the world the ashtray that wasn't worth five dollars. You would think I would have learned from our experiences in other restaurants. At least I learned to enjoy the chaos after the fact. All I remember about that night was Dad's outburst; I don't even remember what I was celebrating.

———⁙———

My father also experienced name substitution. To be more precise, he started calling Nora "Christina" during our visits. I reasoned that since he usually had trouble remembering who Nora was, he just substituted the last female name he had heard. That's when I noticed him squinting at Nora/Christina. "Dad, where are your glasses?"

"I don't wear glasses," he said. I went and asked a staff member about the missing glasses.

"I'm sorry, Dr. Trujillo, but he broke them and threw them away." Great. At least this time they didn't fall in the toilet. *No matter,* I thought, *I'll just wait until next week and take him to get a new pair.*

Having lifted Dad's suspension, the Little School took a field trip. Since he wasn't wearing his glasses, my dad misread the steps on the van as he was getting off. He fell down and hit his head on the curb. The impact gave him a huge gash on his forehead and knocked him unconscious. The bus driver freaked out, called the paramedics and then the home, and the home called me.

When they called they said, "Don't get scared, nothing serious, but your father fell. He has a little bump on his head and had to be taken to the emergency room."

"Nobody gets taken to the emergency room for just a little bump on the head! What happened?"

"Well, you know he threw away his glasses, right? Well, he couldn't see so well, and he fell off the bus."

"Did he hurt himself?"

"Well, he was bleeding a lot . . . and he was unconscious for some time."

"How long?" I asked, imagining massive trauma and blood everywhere.

"Uh, we're not really sure, but by the time the paramedics arrived, he had regained consciousness and was on all fours searching for his glasses."

"So, which emergency room did they take him to?"

"Uh, I don't know."

Here we go again. Find someone to cover for me, call the ERs in the area. Find the hospital and get down there. By then the doctors had already cleaned and sutured the wound, and Dad was sitting on a stretcher. The poor thing looked so lonely sitting there, his shirt all bloody, looking around like he didn't know where he was. When he saw me he had the biggest smile, "Oh good! You came to take me home."

"Pop, you can't go home."

"Oh yes; I'm leaving."

"No, no, no, Dad, I don't know what's going on here. Let me talk to the doctor and find out."

The doctor explained that they had stitched him up to stop the bleeding; but they had ordered some X-rays to make sure he didn't have a fracture in his skull, and they would probably need a CT scan of his brain. At this point I went back to Dad to explain the situation and told him not to worry because I would stay with him. His response was, "Can I have a cigarette?"

"What? They're not going to let you smoke in here."

"Just sneak one in."

"See these oxygen tanks? The sick people? You can't do that."

That got him upset. So of course he took it out on me. He wasn't screaming or struggling. Rather, he pouted as small children do to show you they're upset. He started mumbling angrily in my general direction. I wouldn't take him home, wouldn't give him a cigarette; the hospital people wouldn't let him walk, and one of them even had the audacity to try to put him in a wheelchair! I calmly ignored his grouching and just stayed with him.

Dad was conscious and his vital signs were stable, so he was no longer an emergency. The ER, being the ER, kept getting busy trying to take care of other emergencies. The X-ray department was doing all the emergencies first; it would take care of Dad whenever it got a chance. That was it; he'd had enough. "I'm going outside to smoke, and then I'm going home."

"Do you know how to get home?"

"Nope, but you're driving me."

"No, you're staying until the doctor says you can leave."

When you find yourself in those moments when your mom or dad won't listen to you, you have to find someone they will listen to. I called Robert and asked him, "Listen, baby, can you come over to the hospital? Dad is a little out of it." While I was making the phone call, my dad got up from the stretcher and tried to walk away. However, he got dizzy and would have fallen again if I hadn't caught him. Even he realized that wasn't good. So he stayed on the stretcher until Robert arrived, and that helped keep Dad calm.

After a while Dad started looking at us funny. "Is something wrong, Dad?"

"I have to get up."

"No, you can't. It's only for a little bit longer."

"No, I really need to go."

"You can't go anywhere; you get dizzy."

Then Robert chimed in, "Do you need to pee?" Dad didn't say a word but nodded yes to Robert. He wanted to pee. Once again, since Robert was in the room, I was outranked.

"Pop, you can't walk to the bathroom. Stay here; I'll get a urinal from the nurse." I went to the nurse while keeping one eye on him. I came back with the urinal; he looked at me and said, "Not in front of you. You're my daughter."

"Pop, I'm a doctor."

"I don't care; I am not going to pee in front of you. I'm going to the bathroom."

"No, no, no, no. Please, please just stay put. You use this urinal by sliding your . . ." And he held onto the bed sheets so that I couldn't put the urinal in place. Even though he had Alzheimer's, he still had his pride, and he was not about to let his daughter see his genitals. All this time my boyfriend was on the other side of the curtain till I finally said, "Robert, would you mind coming in here and giving me a hand?"

And I heard from out there, "Oh no, that's your problem."

I insisted, "Please, come in—and I mean now!"

Robert entered with a groan, and my Dad looked at him and then at me. "OK, get out."

"What?"

"If I can't go to the bathroom and I have to pee in this thing, you can't be here. Now get out."

So I went outside the curtain and left Robert alone, which I know Robert must have appreciated. I waited and waited. After a while I heard, "Where is it?"

"I don't know."

"I can't find it. Stick your hand in there."

"I'm not sticking my hand in there."

"But I cannot find it!"

"What's going on in there?" I asked Robert. "Is there a problem?"

"We can't find the hole."

That only confused me more. "What hole?"

"The hole in his underwear."

Dad chimed in, "I'm peeing on myself. Hurry up!"

I stuck my head in and Robert gave me that what-did-you-get-me-into look and said, "He put his underwear on backwards." He turned to my dad and said, "You have to take off your pants and your underwear."

"Not with her looking!" I closed the curtain again and just listened in to Robert grouching as he took off my dad's pants and underwear. Then there was a brief moment of silence till I heard my dad say, "OK, grab it."

"Hell no! That's where I draw the line, Old Man! I'll hold the urinal; you hold your own penis!" I don't know why Robert was upset over the whole thing; personally, I was cracking up on the other side of the curtain. Then, of course, there came the noises that we don't need to explain. But the surprising part was Robert's reaction. "Wow, he really needed to go; this thing is overflowing."

Now that that was all taken care of, I asked Dad about the backward underwear. "Dad, the staff at the home is supposed to help you get dressed in the morning."

"I don't let them in the room. What would your mother think if she knew women were trying to put on my underwear? I'll put it on myself, thank you."

It was extremely irritating when Dad would only listen to Robert. Don't get me wrong, Robert was super sweet. No matter what the crisis, all I had to do was call and he'd be there. But where did he get off becoming my dad's best buddy? I went through the painstaking process of patiently and calmly explaining everything to my dad, and all Robert did was to come in at the last minute and just say what he wanted done, and Dad immediately did it! For some reason no one else in my family seemed upset about this.

As we were walking out of the hospital after this last incident, I couldn't stand it anymore. "Does he talk to you like you're from the old times?"

Robert looked at me, befuddled. "What?"

"I need to know. Does he think you're the Robert he used to work with? Did he know your dad? Is it just a guy thing; is he tired of listening to women?" In response to what I'm sure must have sounded like insane rambling, Robert answered as eloquently as any blindsided man would.

"Huh?"

"Why is it that *my* father does whatever *you* tell him to?"

"Oh, cigarettes."

"I'm sorry, can you repeat that? I . . . I must have heard you wrong."

"Cigarettes. I give him cigarettes."

"You're not supposed to give him cigarettes! They're bad for him! He has COPD! Even the doctor told him he couldn't smoke anymore!"

And in his classic calm manner, Robert smiled devilishly, "That's why he wants them."

Cigarettes. That's all it took. OK, maybe I overcomplicated things. All right, if I had known I could have gotten Dad to comply with me in exchange for cigarettes, I would have sat here proudly proclaiming how clever I was. But that's how it feels when you've been the main caregiver, struggling for years, and someone else comes along and handles things with the greatest of ease. As much as I hated it at that moment, sometimes you have to swallow your pride and let someone else help even if that person is a big clown.

One trick to deal with memory loss is . . . well, to trick the Germans. Do not always try to reason or argue; the whole point is to get them to where they need to be, like when you give a child a lollipop for going to the doctor. Resorting to a little bribery is OK.

I'm sure you can think of a variety of (legal) delights to capture your German's attention. Food, maybe candy, money, material possessions, polka music—anything else they really like. A piece of advice: avoid alcohol. It has a nasty habit of interacting badly with medications. Check with your doctor about whether small doses are OK. Just remember: all good things in moderation. In my Dad's case, a good bribe was cigarettes. And I know that as a doctor I'm supposed to tell you smoking is bad for you, but honestly, Dad had been smoking since he was eight! (Vastly inappropriate, I know). Considering that he had schizophrenia, Alzheimer's, and a variety of other health issues and was already seventy, who cared anymore? It was more important at this stage to just get him to sit still for the doctor. Of all the vices out there, smoking was the least of evils.

At the same time, smoking did have a negative impact on his health, so I didn't want him to be lighting up all the time. So Robert and I started playing good cop, bad cop. Whenever a situation arouse where Dad might be agitated, I would allow Robert to bribe him with one cigarette. Robert always made it a point to remind Dad that he wasn't supposed to be giving him the cigarette and to make sure not to tell me. This increased the value of that one cigarette. Dad "knew" that I wouldn't allow him to smoke and that Robert was taking a risk in giving him this cigarette. "All things in moderation" should be your guideline for bribery. Small amounts of anything will do the least damage and make that item all the more valued.

Bribery

Here's a story to show you the value of bribery. I took Dad, Robert, and Nora on a family outing to the same Italian restaurant where Dad had the incident with the belt. When I saw Dad getting a little agitated, I got the pack of cigarettes from my jacket and handed them to . . . where was Robert? Oh no, he went across the street to look at the wooden fish in the store window. I couldn't give Dad his smokes; I was the bad cop. On the off chance that this would turn out like the dentures (one of those things that Dad never forgot) he would no longer take it seriously when I forbade him to smoke. That only left Nora, the teenager with the ultra-PC, save-the-world hippie teacher, who had been complaining about her grandfather's smoking since she was eight.

I had no choice; I couldn't let Dad drop his pants in the same place twice. Giving the pack to Nora, I told her, "Look, I know you don't like smoking, but Grandpa is a little antsy. So I want you to pretend that you two are sneaking away from me and let him smoke one cigarette." And she did it. Wonder of wonders, there was no lecture about the ills of the tobacco companies. She played the part perfectly. They even made sure that I was distracted on my cell phone so that I wouldn't see him smoking. Of course I wasn't talking to anyone on my cell; I was really watching them through the reflection of the restaurant window. I was so impressed by Nora's ability to just let her grandfather be himself. Dad, being a good grandfather, did tell her that she shouldn't be smoking—not because she was underage but because she was a girl. Girls shouldn't smoke because it's bad for them. And she responded calmly that she didn't smoke but that the pack of cigarettes she was carrying belonged to Robert, who had instructed her to give him one in secret.

When I saw that Dad had finished his cigarette, it was time for the bad cop to bust onto the scene. "I smell smoke. You were smoking, weren't you, Pop?"

And Dad shook his head. "No! No, China. I was just here talking to Nora about . . ."

And Nora picked up for him when he got stuck. "Cars. We were talking about cars."

"Yes, the cars! I was telling her about the cars in the parking lot." I was so proud that Nora had finally learned to not contradict or correct her grandfather. She had even picked a simple, concrete subject: the cars that were right in front of him. She was really enjoying this little game. She had learned to make her visits more enjoyable for everyone by avoiding conflict.

And Dad was very adamant in his cover story. He looked down. "Why, look at all the cigarette butts on the ground. A lot of people were smoking here. That must be what you are smelling."

I was so proud I decided to wrap it up so we could eat a celebration feast. "Good thing you were talking about cars because the doctor already said no more smoking for you."

"That's not true," Dad said suddenly. *Uh oh, this can't be good.* "Dr. Vega said I could smoke four cigarettes a day." Then it hit me that Vega was Robert's last name. Just in time, Robert showed up to the fray with a bag of wooden fish decals. "You told my father that he could smoke four cigarettes a day?"

Robert looked at Dad. "You sold me out."

I continued berating Robert in English. "I'm not really mad! But I'm going to talk loudly to you and poke you like this because I want Dad to think we are fighting over his smoking! I just don't want him to think smoking is OK! Let him think that you're taking a risk by giving him cigarettes!" Even as I explained myself, Robert clutched his bag of dime store decorations to his chest as if I were about to take them away from him.

"Well, I think your dad only wanted you to fight with me as a distraction because Nora just gave him another cigarette. Why don't you yell at her now?"

"I think I'm just going to keep yelling at you! I'm so proud of her! You should have seen her! But please let me know when he finishes that cigarette because I don't want her giving him a third one!"

Chapter 16

Pets and Other Problems

Dealing with my patients gave me insight into issues I didn't face with my own father. Maybe some of these issues are relevant in your life. There are little things that you don't always think about when a major illness comes up. With Alzheimer's, the first things that come to mind are medicines, doctors, health care, etc. The last thing you would think about is a puppy or the car.

Driving

Driving with Alzheimer's: simple—don't do it. It doesn't matter if they don't want to stop driving; it doesn't even matter if they are still driving well. Eventually, the mental deficits are going to catch up to them, and one of the worst places to have an episode is behind the wheel of two tons of steel going forty miles an hour. Germans can get confused and end up getting lost, running red lights, or driving into a farmer's market. Maybe all they need is supervision. Right, because you want to be in the seat next to them when they crash into the Laundromat. Take the keys away.

Pets

Pet therapy is becoming increasingly popular. Therapy dogs offer loving interaction and nonthreatening stimuli. Trainers accompany the dogs to ensure that patients benefit from the interaction. Pet therapy can be very helpful—anyone who has a dog or cat can tell you about the joys of pet love. We didn't have any animals in the house when my father developed Alzheimer's. My mother very wisely concluded that there was no way she could look after a child, a German, and a puppy all at the same time. This was a great disappointment to Nora, who always brought home every lost or injured critter she came across.

I've had Alzheimer's patients who have loved and cared for their pets, even providing better care for their pets than for themselves. I know of one dog that had health insurance when the owner didn't! But as Alzheimer's progresses, Germans start to lose the capacity to care for a pet's needs. For patients who live alone, a pet could be a risky situation or even a dangerous one if the pet is not well trained. If the pet soils the floor, a German may slip and fall because he is not paying attention to these details. Also, animal behavior ranges from perfect to totally bad. Perhaps a German has a guard dog or a big dog for protection and forgets to feed it, leading the dog to become aggressive. Or she might have a dog that's aggressive to strangers, and she forgets to close the door, allowing the dog to get out. And then there are situations you never expect.

I recall one patient who had an adorable little dog. When her children came to visit, they noticed the little fuzzy friend that always followed Mom around wasn't there. They started asking, "Where's Pom-Pom?" When my patient realized the dog had disappeared, she became very distraught. No one had visited her for a week, so her dog's absence had gone unnoticed. Everyone started looking all over the house and the neighborhood.

After some time searching for the dog, I got a call from this patient's terrified son. "She froze Pom-Pom! She put the dog in the freezer!" I dropped my pen in shock. He nervously told me about how his mother was hysterical at having lost her beloved Pom-Pom and how everyone was looking for this dog. Her son went to get her a glass of water to calm her down. He found Pom-Pom when he went to get the ice. "Mom was the only one in the house. I mean, I opened the door, the freezer door. Pom-Pom had her little teeth out! She put her in there alive!"

"OK, OK, calm down. Does Mommy know?"

"No. We haven't told her yet. Dr. T, how do I tell my mom that she froze Pom-Pom?"

At this point I realized that the son needed more treatment than the mom, who wouldn't remember what happened.

There was no point in telling her. Even if her son did tell her the truth, I knew she would forget—but for a while she would suffer horribly for something she really did not mean to do. My treatment was geared more toward the son. "Did you take the dog out of the freezer?"

"Yeah, yeah. What do I do with it?"

"Take it to the backyard and bury it. Put it in a bag. Just get rid of it without your mother seeing it. It's about time we start to talk about the same topic I know you don't want to hear. It's time for Mom not to be by herself. She is good; she is proud; she wants to remain independent. She says, 'Over my dead body because this is my house, and nobody is taking me to a nursing home.' But maybe start thinking of a caretaker. Someone to supervise the cooking and cleaning and do some of the things around the house. To protect her from herself; she doesn't mean to hurt anyone."

"Should . . . should I get her another dog?"

"I think not, for the sake of the pet."

I believe the son ended up telling his mother that she had probably left the door open and Pom-Pom ran away. If your German has a pet, you will have to supervise that pet as well as the German. Otherwise, give the pet to someone else. Keep in mind people can get very attached to pets. It might be difficult to take away your German's companion.

Please don't be horrified by this case. I don't want anyone to be struck with fear at such a story even though I know of several similar instances (not always with a dog). I have five dogs, and I wouldn't want anything like that to happen to them. The point is not to be scared—it is to be educated.

You may think it was odd that we chose not to tell the patient about her dog. But telling her would have been detrimental when she really didn't need to know. If a major event occurs that's directly related to the patient, it is my duty as a doctor to inform the patient and the primary caretaker; so if that's you, you need to understand this. Dead dog, damaged car—not major issues. Surgery—major issue. If there's a medical complication, death in the family, or other major problem, tell them, just don't retell them. If they don't remember the first time, they're going to forget the second time around.

For example, I've had families come to me and say, "Our mom just died. We don't know if we should tell Dad. His mind is already so far gone." My opinion is that patients have a right to know, but if they're not going to understand or if they're frail and it could be harmful to their health, don't say anything. I had another patient whose daughter was very upset. "Every time I visit him, he keeps asking where my mother is, and it always breaks his heart when I have to explain to him that she's been dead for ten years." My answer to that is, "That's simple then: don't tell him! If he keeps forgetting, why are you going to remind him? Tell him she's at the grocery store, she went to Disneyland, she's visiting her cousin in Wyoming—it doesn't matter; either way he'll forget by tomorrow." The point is their minds are not working like yours, so don't kill yourself trying to correct them. Let it go.

Housing

We've already discussed nursing homes and ALFs, but what do you do if the German owns a home? Pom-Pom's owner was very proud like my father. All her life she worked and saved and got herself a house. That was her home and no one was getting her out of it. Her children, like myself and many other children of Alzheimer's patients, didn't want to put her in a home. But as her condition got worse, they had to do something. Like me, they could not provide twenty-four-hour supervision, but she didn't want to live with any of them. She wanted her house! And she interpreted any efforts to place her somewhere else as her children trying to take her house away from her. That wasn't true. But it is understandable why Germans might feel that way. All their lives they've worked and provided and been the head of the family. Now they're old and sick, and here come all these relatives saying "You've got to live in a home." Plus, consider the fact that they probably don't remember the incidents that have caused you so much concern—all those times they've wandered off or left cigarettes burning on the kitchen table—so they don't see any real reason why they need constant care. It feels like you're ganging up on them. To them it really feels like, "You want to get me out of the way because you want my stuff!" Just try to understand that.

All the same, what do you do with a house? It depends on your situation. This particular family, I believe, went with a home companion, a stay-in-home maid. I know some families where the German was still paying for the mortgage and the family found it more affordable to sell the house and use the money to pay the rent in a retirement community. And yes, there are those who, after putting their German in assisted living care, kept the house. Contrary to how it may look, people who do that are not always motivated by greed. There can be a dozen other factors involved. I'm telling you this example so that you don't feel bad if you have to place your German in assisted care. It's not a moral measuring scale that you can look upon and say, "At least I'm not like those creeps. I put mine in a home for the right reasons." There are no "right" reasons, only necessary reasons. These necessities may be medical or financial—or "I don't want him wandering off and accidentally joining a revolution." Alzheimer's is a disease that brings up a lot of emotions in everyone. These emotions will affect treatment.

Chapter 17

Emotions

I t's a lie when people advise you not to let emotions influence caretaking decisions. The only reason you would even care about these decisions is that you have an emotional attachment. I think those who like to give this advice simply mean not to make decisions when you're blinded by extreme emotions like love, hope, guilt, or fear.

Don't let your reaction to Alzheimer's be ruled by fear. Fear makes you of no use to anyone, including yourself. When you start asking yourself questions like "Will she end up forgetting me?" or "What are the chances that I'll get it?" or "Can we afford treatment?" or "How much longer will he live?" worry will naturally set in. But worries are just like that statistic about the twenty-six million cases of Alzheimer's;

they're all valid but you really only need to deal with one. All those fears about what might happen in the future—just grab them, crumple them up, and toss them out. And you can tell that to your German too. Deal with the problems as they come.

You want to prepare for the future; that's OK. There is a difference between planning and worrying. Worrying is thinking of every worst-case scenario. Planning is thinking of every worst-case scenario and what actions should be taken in each case. Planning, you sit down and do purposefully. Worrying, you do all the time.

As you have seen, I took the planning route. Yes, I made a few mistakes. I'm not afraid to admit it. That's the reason I wrote this book: so you can skip over the mistakes I made. From now on, you will never hand a hammer and a chisel over to a German. That's not to say you won't make your own mistakes. When that happens, do the same thing I did: deal with them, laugh about them, and sit down and revise your plans.

The reason you don't want to worry is that worry turns you into a scatterbrain. Your brain becomes clouded with all this fear regarding Alzheimer's. Eventually your brain gets the idea that Alzheimer's equals fear. And you really don't want that concept in your brain. Otherwise, every time you look at your German, you'll feel a slight thud in your chest. Your thoughts will have an unclear nervousness to them. You might confuse this feeling with pity. It will become uncomfortable to be in the same room with the German and you won't know why. That's when worrying has poisoned your mind with fear.

And your loved ones will notice. They may not say anything, but they will notice.

This feeling of fear will become more obvious when you feel a sense of relief whenever something pulls you away from the German. If things come up or you're just too tired, you'll skip a visit. Seizing legitimate reasons to miss a visit slowly turns into making up excuses not to see the German. Fear takes control of your emotions.

Eventually fear will turn into guilt. Every minute of every day that you don't visit is time your loved one spends sitting around waiting for you. Visiting is not something you should just blow off because you don't feel like it—because that short amount of time you spend with your German may be the highlight of their week. You'll feel horrible that you haven't visited your dad in three months, so you go with the intention of making it up to him. But Germans are human too. Their feelings will be hurt. If they're losing their memories anyway, why would they want to hold on to the memories of someone who has hurt them? After three months without reinforcing the preexisting bonds, chances are this visit will be more unpleasant than the ones that led you to avoid him in the first place.

It's OK to feel a little worried. It's human to avoid things that frighten us. You're not a bad person if you've ever had these feelings; you're just a scared person. You're human; you've had a weak moment. Let's conquer the fear right now.

What if you've already done the three-month vanishing act? If you didn't care, you wouldn't be reading this book. Don't worry—we can fix it.

Reestablish a Bond

Don't be upset if your parent doesn't remember you. Just take a deep breath and remember the rules of communicating with Germans. Approach them from the front. Identify yourself. "Hello, Mom, it's me, your daughter Suzanne." Also, you can have someone else announce you, usually the primary caretaker. "Good morning, Mr. Brooklowski. I have a big surprise! Your son Arnold came to visit!" The peppy attitude helps. Remember Germans are easily influenced by what's immediately in front of them. So a cheerful attitude will rub off on them. That's not to say that if you go in there all smiles, they won't respond with resentment or obscenities. What do you do then? Run away like you did last time? No, you've made it this far. That was hard enough. Don't give up now. If it gets stuck in their head that you didn't visit, you can apologize and explain yourself. "I'm sorry I haven't seen you in a while; I've been busy with . . ." Or you can be forthcoming: "I'm sorry; you're right—I should have come sooner, but it unnerves me so much knowing that you're sick." The whole point is to get to "I'm here now. I may have fumbled on the way over, but I'm here now." And don't say that unless you really mean it.

Change the Subject

Try talking about something you know they'll like or anything that they are interested in discussing that doesn't relate to your past absence. And you never know— for all your worrying, they may not even remember that they haven't seen you in three months.

Deal with Resentment

Some relatives might disapprove of your lack of involvement. "How can you not go see your own mother? You are just a selfish individual who puts your suffering before the needs of others. The rest of us visit her religiously!"

If you are having such a conflict, you'll just have to work through it. The reason everyone is upset is because they're all scared too. They probably have the same fears and worries, but they're dealing with the issue differently. If you really want to visit, approach them. Share your feelings. Remind them that you're all family and offer to go together as a group. Empty your mind of the idea that you are visiting a sick relative. You're still visiting your father or your mother—they've just changed a little.

Nora

love those bizarre cases. The little blurbs in the newspaper that report "man in coma awakens after forty-six years" or "child's terminal cancer miraculously disappears." It is always so encouraging to read those stories. It hypes you up. Anything is possible. Then I visit Grandpa. And it hits you . . . you're not going to be one of those incredible stories. Like the saying goes, someone is going to win the lottery; it just won't be you. But knowing that has never stopped anyone from playing.

I think everyone holds on to that bit of hope that the person they love will get better. You hope that you'll walk into their room and in a snap they will know who you are even though you know it's not going to happen. There's nothing wrong with wishful hope—it's what drives scientists to find cures. The trick is not to become disappointed when you walk into the room and your loved one doesn't recognize you in a snap. Joy isn't waiting for those magical moments that aren't going to happen. It's finding ways to enjoy the moments that you have.

Chapter 18

Ay, Ay, Ay

After years of successfully treating Alzheimer's patients I started getting a reputation. People began to seek me out with more advanced cases. Eventually some families started coming whose relatives were already in the final stages of Alzheimer's. One patient's caretakers complained, "All she says is 'Ay, ay, ay,' all day long."

"Are you OK?"

"Ay, ay, ay."

"Do you feel fine?"

"Ay, ay, ay."

"Do you need something?"

"Ay, ay, ay." No matter what they asked, the answer was always the same. She just kept repeating that one audible sound all day long. The sense of powerlessness in these situations is overwhelming. Looking at this patient and her family, I felt the same frustration that I had experienced when I first started looking for doctors to explain what was wrong with my father. Part of me was very afraid that this was what Dad would eventually become. With a heavy heart I told the family, "Look, there's really nothing that can be done. I'm sorry, but once they reach this stage, they're not going to regain any function." It was like telling them the words I was afraid of hearing, to which their response was, "Oh, we know, Doc. We just want you to make her shut up."

Oh, man! I was simultaneously shocked and relieved! It left a big impression on me that this family had such reasonable expectations. *Can you get her to shut up?* Some out there might find their request insensitive. Let me tell you, after you spend eight or twelve hours listening to this *ay, ay, ay,* it gets extremely annoying to say the least. So I wanted to see what caused this behavior.

Patients in the last stages of Alzheimer's are known as being in Stage 6 or Stage 7, which originally was Stage 4 and is now considered likely to be Stage 3. I avoided listing the stages of Alzheimer's in this book for two reasons. First, they've changed a few times, and I'm still unsure if the stages will be revised again in the future. Currently there are three recognized stages: mild, moderate, and severe. Second, I don't want you developing stage fright; you don't need a list to tell you that your loved one is going to get worse. You'll notice when they get worse. Instead, I affectionately gave in to calling these the "Ay, Ay, Ay" patients.

Most of the time, as they get to the later stages of the disease, patients grow more detached from the outside world. There is not only memory loss but also loss of muscle function and brain capacity. Patients may not be able to walk and may even have difficulty moving. They lose their ability to speak, becoming unable to communicate. The frustration simply grows when some of these patients who can't talk only scream. That's when it hit me. *That's it! They're acting out* because *they can't talk.*

If your child throws a temper tantrum and you try to ignore it, after five minutes you tell that kid "Shut up!" and you manage to stop them or entertain them. Now you have this adult who's going at it. How long can you ignore this "Ay, Ay, Ay"? It's very difficult to get used to. You can't ignore them because they're not going to get bored, and even if they do, they'll forget they're bored. You can't spank them; it's not going to work. Don't think of these behaviors as childish— think baby. Let's learn an advanced German speaking lesson. In the Ay, Ay, Ay stage it's not so much about talking as it is about listening. Again, Ay, Ay, Ay patients have mostly lost their capacity for regular speech. Ergo, instead of verbalizing, they express themselves through their actions.

Between early life and late life there are some similarities. Some refer to old age as the second childhood. Let me show you the comparison. If you were sick as a baby, you would cry your eyes out. It might have been just an earache, but a baby can't say, "Mommy, my ear hurts." Likewise, the Ay, Ay, Ay patient may be screaming bloody murder, and they may just be trying to force out a stool. If you don't feed the baby, the baby can't feed himself. If you don't feed the Ay, Ay, Ay, the Ay, Ay, Ay can't feed himself.

I checked this patient over; there was no medical cause for discomfort. What if it was something simpler? She was clean, fed, and healthy. Why else would a baby cry? Well, she couldn't walk and had lost a good deal of brain function; maybe her mind was seeking stimuli.

The first and best approach in trying to create stimuli is to give Alzheimer's patients something that will keep them entertained. Don't try the TV. Patients can't keep up with the loud noises and constant changes on TV. They may not be able to understand the program or follow a storyline, so trying to watch a TV show might create more confusion. They need something more physical. Some concrete object that will keep their hands busy is a better option.

Dolls

Find dolls with little cloth dresses, bright colors, or something that will catch their attention. Perhaps you've walked into a nursing center and seen this. Nurses figured out to give Alzheimer's patients dolls. There is an instinct of play. And even if they pick at little things or throw the dolls away, they are still responding to the stimulus. Remember, you are dealing with someone in a geriatric chair who once played with toys in a baby chair. At this stage the functions are not exactly the same, but the behaviors seem to be similar. Just like children, Alzheimer's patients will put these toys in their mouths. Make sure there are no small parts they can swallow, so no Barbies—stick to big huggable dolls or other such toys.

In the case of my first Ay, Ay, Ay patient, that was all she needed—a simple form of entertainment, a nonthreatening stimulus that she could focus on. That was it! Then I got to thinking. What else could cause these behaviors in patients with advanced Alzheimer's? As I have stated, you can't forget the human factor. Just because they have Alzheimer's doesn't mean Alzheimer's is the problem. Other conditions can occur in older people.

I started applying what I had learned to patients who came in with "aggressive" or "violent" behavioral problems. These were the Ay, Ay, Ay patients who got very nasty. Not only would they scream, but they would also bite, spit, and hit you if they could. They weren't interested in dolls or any stimuli. Something else was troubling them.

"Where does it hurt?"

"Ay . . . Ay . . . Ay."

"Point with the finger."

"Ay . . . Ay . . . Ay."

All they do is look at you or look away from you, and if you try to point to certain parts of their body they slap your hand away. Then it dawned on me that many times, patients were suffering from other conditions that agitated their Alzheimer's. Would treating any medical condition stop the Ay, Ay, Ay? Not necessarily. Maybe yes, maybe no; but there might be something else that is causing the aggressive behavior other than the Alzheimer's itself. What really surprised me was that most of the time these behaviors were the result of something really simple. Small things are commonly misdiagnosed and can snowball into something worse. There were three big ones that I noticed. These three things often cause Germans to be misdiagnosed with psychiatric conditions.

A Dirty Little Secret

Most of the time, in a desperate attempt to treat all of their elderly patients' medical conditions, including the psychiatric conditions, doctors concoct all kinds of medical cocktails. These cocktails are meant to control high blood pressure, diabetes, respiratory problems, and other health issues associated with old age. Sometimes the side effects of these medications cause patients to have problems. You'll notice the major ones (like if they turn blue) with no difficulty, but what about a side effect like constipation? A lot of medications, as well as other things, may cause constipation.

Let's face it: no one really likes talking about constipation, so we tend to push it to the back of our minds. When a patient doesn't move the bowels every day or every other day, the caretaker or family may not notice. What happens is an interesting condition called fecal impaction. Feces dry up in their guts, and after a while, they get fecal matter all the way from their rectum to the beginning of their colon. These patients feel constipated or bloated. You yourself would not feel like eating anything. However, this eighty-four-year-old individual with Alzheimer's cannot tell you, "I'm bloated, I'm uncomfortable, and I don't want to eat. I have not pooped in a week." In the first place, they don't remember; in the second, they don't know how to explain themselves because by this stage all of their capacity to speak is gone. And here you come with a plate of food because what is the norm? People need to eat.

They're old, frail, and in this wheelchair or geriatric chair and haven't eaten anything for two days, and here you are insisting that they eat. Bam! There goes the tray; there goes the food; and you're running and crying and all upset if you're a family member. If you're a caretaker, you're all fed up. They get sent to the hospital for aggressive behavior, throwing things, and pushing you away. You tell the doctor, "Doctor, she doesn't want to eat." The doctor comes and gives medication to enhance the appetite or to control the aggressive behavior.

The problem is they are full of dried-up feces, which by now don't move very well. And they are not going to get out unless you get your German to the hospital and some doctor picks up on the fact that maybe the aggressive behavior is the German's way of saying, "I don't know how to tell you this, but the fact is I don't want to eat anything because I'm constipated. I've been constipated for weeks. I don't want to eat, and here you come with a plate of food. And you should know by now that I'm not moving my bowels, and here's the plate to your face." Bam! And even though they have been having some minor bowel movements, they still have this fecal impaction that is bloating them.

Sometimes the doctor can pick up on that, especially a doctor who specializes in Alzheimer's. However, a lot of times patients get admitted through the emergency room or sent to the psychiatric department. In the psychiatric department they are going to look for psychiatric problems: altered mental status elderly patient with dementia of the Alzheimer's type, aggressive behavior, refusing to eat, refusing to take medications. And they get sent to the inpatient services at the hospital, where someone thinking it's only appetite or aggression will try to prescribe more medications that cause more dry bowels and constipation; and the patient is still not eating.

If you have some experience, you may want to order something called a KUB, which is an X-ray of the abdomen, and in a very large percentage of the cases, you find that, "Oh boy, no wonder this patient was aggressive. If you came close to my face with a plate of food and I had so much feces in my guts, I'd throw the plate in your face too." The treatment is to disimpact the patient. There are laxatives, but if they don't work, the extremely upsetting, painful, and even embarrassing recourse is for a nurse to put on gloves. What you have at the end is a smiling patient who goes, "Ay, Ay, Ay." Not because they feel bad but because they feel good, but they don't know how to tell you. And then they eat without doctors having to give them medication. "I threw that plate at your face because I was full of feces. Now I'm not, so I can eat. I can feel better."

Is the aggressive behavior really part of the Alzheimer's complex or part of the body's natural processes that are not functioning, perhaps because of all the medical treatments or other aging problems? That's an important point to find out.

Dirty Secret Two Is Number One

Other times when you find Alzheimer's patients becoming aggressive and developing all kinds of really weird or bizarre behaviors in which they get aggressive, confused, disoriented, withdrawn, and so forth, the cause may be a urinary tract infection. What happens is some of these patients can no longer hold their urine and have little accidents. So what have we developed in our creative society? Big boys' and girls' diapers. Now children are more active, while most of these Ay, Ay, Ay patients just sit in this pee, sometimes for hours. It is not as easy as with a baby where you just stick a finger into the diaper and say, "Oh, it's wet." Try doing that with an elderly person. Try to check the diaper of someone who is thinking, "Why are you trying to touch my privates?" They'll get defensive. So you only change them when they go to bed or not as often as is necessary. What happens is the urine sits there, bacteria grows, and sometimes the patients defecate, and that goes up the urinary tract. And voilà, you have a urinary tract infection.

Urinary tract infections (UTIs) don't tend to produce symptoms you would typically associate with infection, such as fever. "Mom is real hot. She has a fever. She must have an infection somewhere." UTIs don't tend to give you fever, but from my personal experience, these infections will cause patients to show erratic behavior. They don't feel right; something inside them is wrong but they don't know what, and they respond with out-of-control behavior.

Again, the patient is sent to the hospital and the psychiatry department. The doctors are looking to control the behavior so that the patient can safely return to their regular environment. Here you are again thinking it's behavior and looking for behavior treatments. Getting a urine culture and sensitivity has yielded a very large percentage (in my personal experience, more than sixty percent of the time) of cases in which this altered mental status and aggressive behavior of elderly Alzheimer's patients is caused by a urinary tract infection, which gets nicely treated with an antibiotic. After treatment, the patient's behavior goes back to normal.

Thirsty for Dirty Secret Number Three

Alzheimer's patients have a very hard time moving around and reaching the fridge and the water pitcher or the water fountain. Why? Because even if they're thirsty and they start moving toward it, by the time they get close they forget they went there to drink some water.

Dehydration is another bad issue for these patients. The body is 70 percent water and requires a certain amount of water for its function to be maintained as healthily as possible. The problem is that every single medication that any doctor prescribes has been researched on people who are fully hydrated. If patients forget to drink water, all of a sudden the concentration of the dose is probably a lot higher than it should be. So if you're dehydrated, you're going to have a lot more of the side effects of these medications. Also, these medications are going to have a very hard time exiting the body once they're metabolized, so these meds are leaving residual traces that start building up. In addition to that, many of these Alzheimer's patients already have cardiac problems or high blood pressure. And what is the treatment? A water pill. A water pill dries you up a little bit so that your heart can function better.

Lack of water causes chaos inside the body, leading to behavioral problems because the body is trying to convey the message that something is wrong to an outside world that no longer understands this individual. And we don't pick up on these signals. Something as simple as monitoring fluid intake can avoid all that.

The other side of that coin is human behavior. In many care situations it is best not to give patients a lot of water because they pee a lot, and that means a lot of diaper changes and laundry over soiled clothes and sheets. If your seven-year-old wets the bed, the first thing the pediatrician will say is, "No water after 6 p.m." You give your child less water so that she will not wet the bed because you are tired of washing sheets or putting the mattress outside to dry.

Keeping regular bathroom habits is part of our everyday lives, but Ay, Ay, Ay patients have trouble taking care of these needs. Their caretakers might be overwhelmed. They may have too many patients, so it is very difficult to keep all of these people hydrated. And what are you going to do, give a daily or weekly blood test to all of these people to check if their water is depleted? Are you going to get an X-ray of their abdomens to make sure they are not impacted? Are you going to get a sample of urine every week and test it? No. But pay attention because changes in their behavior may not necessarily be the Alzheimer's itself or the worsening of the disease making them aggressive. It might be the way they're trying to convey the message: "Ay, ay, ay, something is wrong but I can't tell you what it is." These Ay, Ay, Ay's, the cries or the behavioral changes, are an attempt to get those desperate feelings out when patients can no longer express them verbally. When these symptoms are misidentified as behavior problems, patients lose the chance to receive care at an appropriate facility. Instead, they get rushed to psychiatric hospitals, and then we totally miss the problem, add more medications, and send them right back with the same thing, simply saying, "It's Alzheimer's; it's getting worse. That's the way it goes." There are a number of things that will happen to these patients that they can't express. These are three simple things that you need to keep in mind.

Rule of Thumb

Now how can you tell the problem is one of the Dirty Secrets and not just the Alzheimer's getting worse? The rule of thumb is to stop and consider whether your loved one's behavior has totally changed within a few days. If a patient's condition has been at a plateau for a while and within two to four days he suddenly starts to act out, chances are something is bothering him—either the Dirty Secrets or something else.

Other factors may cause an unknown irritation. Arthritis, a headache, an allergy, sinus pressure, a rash, or even the annoying music coming from the next room. It may be that your loved one is feeling arthritic pain on this very cold day. Meanwhile, you're insisting, "Mom, get up from the chair. Let's go watch some TV." Mom doesn't want to move. She can't tell you, "Just leave me alone. I'm hurting." These patients can no longer tell you verbally about the things that affect them. They can't tell you what's hurting, so they start acting out. So consider the minor afflictions they had before they entered the Ay, Ay, Ay stage and other ailments not uncommon in the elderly. Keep that in mind.

Dirty Little Secret Four

What other medical complications may cause Alzheimer's symptoms to worsen? There is one other thing I have observed in my own patients, the fourth dirty little secret. I am not going to claim that I am an expert on hypertension or on the control of high blood pressure. But in my experience, this is what I've found out. Seniors have a lot of plaque in their bloodstreams as well as their brains. Plaque builds up over the years for various reasons. The plaque in the blood vessels is part of the reason why blood pressure normally goes up as we age. Blood is responsible for transporting oxygen to every cell of the body. The body raises the blood pressure to force the blood through this clogging vessel to get some blood to every single organ, including the brain, and maintain the body's vitality. We normally say we know high blood pressure is definitely not good. It will damage those same vessels, even though this is apparently a normal reaction to get blood to the organs. So we try to lower the blood pressure. It is not unusual to find elderly Alzheimer's patients with a blood pressure of ninety over sixty. And when he wasn't ill, before he needed treatment, this same individual's blood pressure was 120 over eighty. Now we expect his blood to get to all the vital organs at almost half of the pressure. What happens is what we call hypoxia: a decreased amount of oxygen getting to the brain.

Taking oxygen away from any healthy human causes hallucinations, behavioral changes, confusion, and disorientation. In fact, if the brain doesn't get any oxygen for a period of three to five minutes, you will have brain damage. We tend to treat elderly patients' blood pressure aggressively. We're very happy when blood pressure is low. And I'm not advocating stopping treatment for hypertension; some patients have three, four, or five different antihypertensive medications that are clinically indicated and necessary. But try to maintain the blood pressure within a relatively decent level so that enough oxygen gets to the brain to avoid a degree of confusion. Perhaps a dose adjustment might be sufficient.

Another problem is that seniors who are confused and disoriented and are still a little bit on the ambulatory side have a much higher possibility of falling. At this age, they will probably be suffering from osteoporosis. Their bones are going to be very brittle. If these patients fall, bones are going to break much more easily. Some medications may cause osteoporosis as well, but there are also medications to help with it.

The bones might get some calcium and get a little bit stronger, but the individual needs to get exercise. Sometimes it is very difficult to get these patients to walk around as Alzheimer's progresses and they become more confused and unable to follow directions.

Science and medicine have reached a point at which most conditions can be treated and, if not cured, improved. Let's not forget what I always tell everybody: the human factor. If you don't understand what may be causing a new behavior, consider the possibility that maybe it doesn't necessarily require a pill. It might be something very simple to solve. In my experience, if behavior has been at a plateau and all of a sudden it gets worse within a span of a few days, look at non-Alzheimer's–related conditions because the patient is much like a baby who can't tell you what he's feeling and may require medical care of a simple nature. What happens when these elderly patients become aggressive and agitated, when they are bothered by something, but doctors can't tell what it is? We tend to medicate them more. You can't remove the human factor.

Nora

I had gotten comfortable with visiting Grandpa on a weekly basis. Of course, he still didn't remember me. In truth, even though I did use some of my mom's teachings, I really didn't say much. I would walk around with him, listen to him, and agree with him when he explained how flags were tablecloths except for the American flag because it was designed by Jesus. Even though he didn't recognize me, visiting Grandpa was still fun. It was relaxing—and very entertaining when he would say or do something that caught others off guard. Mom would be dying of embarrassment, but that only made it more hilarious. Mostly, however, I had fun because we would take Grandpa out to walk around, and I got to choose where we went. If we didn't have any errands to run, we usually ended up at some local shopping center.

On this particular day, however, we did have an errand. Robert needed to stop by Home Depot for some supplies. When we got to the ALF, Grandpa was ready to go. He hugged my mom, "Moraima," slapped my dad on the arm, "Robert," then stared at me . . . "Michelle!" At least this time he confused me for my cousin instead of that annoying television anchor. Anyway, when he heard we weren't going to the mall this time, he rushed out the door. "Don't just stand there; we have construction to do! Let's go! You too, Christina." *Crap, I'm back to being that television chick.*

Since any hardware store is Robert's candy shop, he was even more eager than Grandpa to get to Home Depot. No sooner did we park before Robert started walking on ahead without us. Mom went to catch up to him, so I stayed with Grandpa because he couldn't walk very fast at all. He always had difficulty walking, but he refused to use a wheelchair. Heaven help you if you even hinted at the word "wheelchair."

Grandpa started making his inspired commentary about what he observed. "They walk like a cowgirl and a farmer." I really had no idea what he meant, but I still laughed behind my lips. Then he shouted after Mom and Robert, "Hey, farmer, get back here; Christina can't walk that fast." Of course, I was the slow one. Grandpa was only staying with me because it was the chivalrous thing to do.

Realizing his own lack of parking lot etiquette, Robert came back. "Sorry, Old Man, but come on; we have repairs to do. We need to take care of construction."

I couldn't help myself. "Yeah, farmer, we gotta fix that chicken coop."

Robert just smiled at me and said, "You're right, Christina. Now why don't you go on an' get me that there trolley 'fore some other feller think o' takin' it." As I went to get the hand trolley, I realized I had been set up when I overheard Robert say, "Hey, Old Man, what does she walk like?"

I ignored the joking farmer until all of a sudden I heard my grandfather exclaim, "Damn! Nora has her grandmother's ass!"

Oh my God! Grandpa actually remembered my name. That was the first time in almost ten years that he had recognized me—I mean, really recognized me—without someone helping him. And it was because of my . . . butt.

Moraima

I can explain that. There are two possible explanations.

Unlike dying brain cells, when a memory is forgotten, it isn't necessarily lost forever. Some memories wax and wane as in the case of the dentures or the one time Robert gave Dad permission to smoke four cigarettes a day. For some reason Dad always managed to remember the things I wanted him to forget. This is why some people might believe that a German is faking. Alzheimer's patients may honestly forget something and months later recall it out of the blue. Memories are mysterious in that way. I know of cases where a person had half of his brain removed and still retained his memories.

The other explanation is that even in the late stages of Alzheimer's, the brain is still capable of logical reasoning. Nora didn't use all the lessons I've given you, like repeating her name frequently in conversation, but she did learn to avoid conflict and listen. That alone made her interactions with her grandfather pleasant. I hadn't taught Nora to reinforce her name at that time because I was the one who was constantly reinforcing her identity for Dad. I would put my arm around her and say, "Look, your granddaughter Nora came with me." Or "Here is Nora." And he would acknowledge her and then forget her name after two minutes. And Nora did the right thing; instead of constantly correcting him (and getting frustrated in the process) she went along with it. It didn't matter if he called her Debby, Patty, or even Christina as long as he was good enough to talk.

Even when Dad couldn't recognize Nora, his brain could still process the fact that *I* referred to her as Nora. So looking at this person whom we called his granddaughter and referred to as Nora, he noticed a resemblance to his wife's derriere. Knowing that this was not his wife or one of his daughters (our booties not being that big), Dad concluded of his own logical ability that this was in fact his granddaughter with the big backside—Nora.

If you've ever tried to redo an essay or report that got lost, then you can understand how frustrated your German often feels. You probably forgot exactly what you had written in the original document. But you managed to write a second report. Sometimes it's better the second time around. Then you truly appreciate these moments, these windows in time where you can hold a conversation and it feels like you're talking to the person you've always known as if they aren't sick but have only been away for a while.

Nora

I imagine it must have been like waking up in the middle of your life, like that first cognitive memory. Imagine waking up and seeing a woman you've never seen before but knowing she is your wife. Your wife says, "Isn't it wonderful? Today Jo-Ann graduates." And you go and watch the graduation ceremony. You know where the school is; you know Jo-Ann; and you know who everyone else is even though you've never seen them before. It's as if all your life before you've been sleeping, and now you're waking up from that slumber.

After that moment, Grandpa seemed to remember me. He spent the afternoon asking me questions as we walked around Home Depot, his arm wrapped around my shoulders. Just like Mom, he was a big supporter of education. As we exited the gardening section he started saying, "Nora, soon you have to think about going to college so that you can become a great doctor and heal the world." I think I know where Mom got her educational obsession from.

"I already started college."

"Really! It's good that you skipped the other grades. That shows you are smart. We need smart doctors." Of course I hadn't skipped ahead, but he really didn't register my high school years.

"Actually, Grandpa, I'm studying communications. Specifically, the writing track."

Grandpa didn't like that. Furious, he stepped away from me. "What? No, no, no, no, no, no! Where is your mother? Why did she not stop this?" Just as I thought we were about to have a major incident in the lighting department, Grandpa suddenly calmed down. "Wait, you will become a writer. Will you write about me?"

"Of course."

And he swelled up like a proud rooster. "Then you were very smart to study writing. That way you will know the correct way to tell my story." He put his arm around me once more and continued walking toward plumbing supplies. "Now you will become a famous writer, and everyone will know my story. And my message will spread to the whole world, and then there will be world peace . . ."

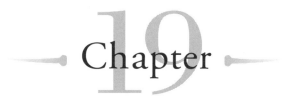

Chapter 19

Disasters

D r. T's number one rule: assume nothing. Just because someone is in an ALF or nursing home doesn't mean that home will be prepared for a major disaster. When I was growing up in the tropics, hurricanes were nothing new. I made sure in advance and in person that Dad's ALF had plenty of supplies, had boarded up all the windows, and was not in an evacuation zone. Hurricane Andrew was the only major storm we went through while Dad was in the ALF, and he was in a safer place than we were. Nora and I were without power for over a month while Dad watched it all on the news in his air-conditioned room.

Fortunately an emergency situation never came up, but if for whatever reason the home couldn't guarantee my dad's safety, I had already included him in my emergency plans. I had a list of all his medications and when he had to take them. I stored extra supplies in case he needed to stay with us. I made sure there would be enough space for him and his things in the car just in case we needed to drive out. You get the idea: make sure to keep the German in your emergency plans even if he or she lives in a care facility. If you are under evacuation orders, take the German with you. But even for all preparations there is always the unforeseen as I discovered one Tuesday in September.

I was working at the Veterans Hospital when I heard. After going through the same shock and fear that everyone else in this country did, I finally remembered, "Oh God, Dad!" I didn't know about the other residents, but I knew my dad. The man was fixated with America and its flag. How would he react if he knew his beloved country was under attack? I called up the home and the employee on the other end of the line was horrified. "Oh, doctor, this is terrible. I just saw on the news."

"Turn off the television!" I yelled at her. "Turn off the television!"

"Oh, none of the patients have seen anything."

"Good, then turn off the television! Do not let them near the television or the radio! Don't let them go outside! Do you understand?" She understood. Such breaking news reports, as troubling as they are to us, would severely agitate anyone with dementia. For the rest of that day there was no television. Instead the ALF treated residents to records of their favorite songs from the old days.

They did a very good job. For every call that they got, they would remind worried family members not to mention what had happened. I myself called at least twice every day. For the next week, the ALF left the television unplugged. The staff was always smiling and cheerful around the patients, distracting them with activities and old-time music. Only when they were sure that no one was around would one of the staff go to the kitchen and turn on the small television set they had hidden to watch the latest news. But for the patients in that home, 9/11 never happened.

⸻

Nora

The fallout from 9/11 kept Mom very busy. She had not been able to visit Grandpa in over two weeks and would not be able to see him this weekend, either. So she asked Robert and me to go for her and take him out. She made it very clear that we were not to tell Grandpa about what had happened and to avoid anything that referred to 9/11. When we got there, Grandpa was very happy to see us. He forgot that he hadn't seen us in two weeks. He did want to know where Mom was.

"Ah, you know how her work is, Old Man," said Robert. "They made her work the weekend."

"That's too bad, but I'm sure she'll come tomorrow."

Since we were supposed to avoid any place where anything about the attacks might be mentioned, Robert reasoned that we should take Grandpa to a Chinese buffet.

Contrary to Robert's assumption, though most of the people in the restaurant were Chinese, they still talked in English and Spanish. Fortunately they were considerate enough not to talk about recent events. After the meal, Grandpa wanted to walk. We pleasantly strolled down the plaza at Grandpa's shuffling pace, which made it easy for me to walk slightly ahead and block any newspaper stands. Anytime we passed people talking about the events, Robert and I would call Grandpa's attention to us so that he wouldn't hear. It was a little nerve-racking. Robert and I were like the Special Ops for Blissful Ignorance.

At the end of the block was a Kmart, and Grandpa wanted to go in. The moment he stepped inside, he was awestruck. Robert and I looked at each other, trying to decide what we should do. There were American flags everywhere. It was like a dream come true for Grandpa. He didn't want to leave. He walked up and down every single aisle looking at all these different flags. Flags on mugs, flags on t-shirts, flags for your car, flags for your car dealership lot, teddy bears with flags, pictures of firemen lifting flags, big flags, little flags. This whole time Robert and I just prayed, *Please don't let him notice what the flags are saying.*

Then we passed a CD display, and of course all the CD covers had pictures of flags. "Hey, Nora, what do they say? All the pictures, what do they say?" All the CDs, like most of the things in the store, were for various charities and relief efforts, but I couldn't tell him that. So I found the one phrase that was on most of these CDs. "They say 'God bless America.'"

I was trying to think of a good story to explain why there would be so many CDs with the same song when I noticed Grandpa's face. He had an expression of what I can only describe as patriotic dignity. His eyes welled up. "I told you. Everyone says I'm crazy, but I told them. And there's the proof. I was right. You see it. Now is when everyone has learned." And he leaned over and whispered in my ear, "See, I'm not as crazy as I let everyone think I am." And for a moment in time he was right. In that Kmart he was a prophet instead of a patient having another incident. "God bless America," he exclaimed. No one was alarmed by his comments; they simply nodded at him with respect.

And for an instant I felt like he wasn't mentally ill at all, that his knowledge was simply more than his own brain could handle, more wisdom than the world was ready for. "Now all we have to do is get a team of doctors, one for every body part—one for the ears, one who specializes in eyes. And we travel with them and we will heal the world. . . ." I still like to think that he was right.

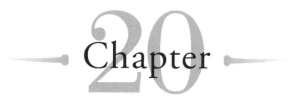

Chapter 20

End

Nora

February 16, 2002, was the day my grandfather, Esmeraldo Trujillo, passed away. My mother took it very hard. Far more so than I, for as sad as I was at that funeral, part of me was very much at peace. I remember seeing Grandpa in his casket and thinking he would sit up at any moment even though I knew that wouldn't happen. As I held my mother while she cried, I couldn't help thinking I should have been more distraught. Just as he finally started to recognize me, he was taken from us. I should have been upset at the unfairness of the situation. But I wasn't. However, I can only feel what I feel. And I did not feel the full force of his loss until later.

As cruel or odd as it may sound, Alzheimer's made it easier to deal with his passing. Most of my life when I talked to my grandfather, it was like he wasn't there; now that he was gone, I found myself still talking to him. It was like when I was a child and Grandpa went to the home and I turned to the invisible part of him that lived in the walls. I felt as if we no longer had to compete with Alzheimer's. Now I could speak to Grandpa and—at least I'd like to believe—he would understand. Now that I no longer had to deal with his sickness, I could keep my happy memories of him. Now he was at peace.

But the biggest solace was when I realized Grandpa's funeral was on President's Day. As we drove down to the cemetery, all the streets were lined with flags, almost like a tribute to him. The funeral procession was filled with many of Mom's coworkers from the hospital to comfort her. Doctors from various fields all came together for my grandfather. He got his wish. And I believe that wherever he was, he knew it and he was happy.

⸺⸻✦⸻⸺

Moraima

It took me a long time to deal with my father's passing. I was lucky that Robert and Nora were there to handle the funeral arrangements because I couldn't handle it. But they were kept so busy attending to everyone and trying to comfort me that they didn't get a chance to grieve. Not a day goes by that I don't still think of him. It was hard when I would wake up Saturday mornings and remember that we couldn't go to visit him anymore. Time was stolen from us, first by his mental illness, then by Alzheimer's, and finally by his passing. Everything reminded me of him. I often found myself having a conversation with him in my mind; I imagined him sharing fatherly words of encouragement that he couldn't tell me when he was sick.

The story of my father's life was full of so many tragedies, triumphs, and twists as to make Charles Dickens look tame. To close his story with Alzheimer's is a sad ending. So I don't view Dad's struggle with Alzheimer's as the end of his story; I view it as just one story in a life rich with many stories. And just as he put a happy spin on all the stories of his life, this one is a comedy—a comedy of errors. And your story, just like Alzheimer's itself, can be a tragedy or a comedy. It all depends on the way it's told.

It happened that I was teaching some residents about dementia of the Alzheimer's type, and I believe I asked for an example of sundowning. A young intern gave me the generic answer of "sleepwalking." I think it was because I was so sensitive at that time that I became upset at such a lousy response. "Sleepwalking? Are you serious? How about waking up in the middle of the night, forgetting the woman in bed is your wife, and accusing her of being a hooker!" The entire group was taken aback by that answer. They started looking at each other until finally one of them said to me, "Dr. T, that's not in the book."

"Oh, of course it's not in the book; that was my father." That little revelation really shocked them; so I continued, "Your textbook isn't going to tell you that they're going to scream at hoochies in the mall or drop their pants at a restaurant. I will give $100 to the person who can find the section in that book that warns you of a risk of your patient wandering off and joining a revolutionary group!" One of them actually started flipping through the pages. "Frank, I was being sarcastic! You're not going to find it in that book. I should penalize you $100 for being that dumb! There is something you are not going to find in your textbooks. It is called the human element." And a funny thing happened; I started telling the stories of all the things my father did . . . and they laughed. That day, my father was able to teach this next generation of doctors things they never knew about Alzheimer's and would never find in their textbooks. And I was happy. I enjoyed remembering all the times my dad did these crazy things that made me want to pull my hair out at the time. And that's really what anyone who really cares for someone with Alzheimer's wants at the end—to be able to look back and laugh, knowing that even when it felt tough, you were there and your loved one's life was better because of it. So is yours.

About the Author

Moraima Trujillo, MD

Moraima Trujillo is a board-certified psychiatrist with over thirty years of experience. Her inspiration to enter the field of psychiatry came from her father, who suffered from schizophrenia and developed Alzheimer's in the last fifteen years of his life. She has devoted her life to treating patients in a variety of facilities—such as community mental health centers, the criminal justice system, crisis intervention units, hospitals, and the veterans administration—and has handled some of the most severe cases. She has also sought to spread her knowledge and experience as a teacher, educating locally, nationally, and internationally about such topics as mental illness, drugs, and HIV/AIDS. She has trained residents in psychiatry at the University of Miami and is involved in research to improve treatments. She lives in Miami and enjoys fishing, just like her father.